Controversies in Transfusion Medicine: Immune Complications and Cytomegalovirus Transmission

Editors

Sanford R. Kurtz, MD
Chairman, Department of Laboratory Medicine
Lahey Clinic Medical Center
Burlington, Massachusetts

Michael L. Baldwin, MBA, MT(ASCP)SBB
Blood Bank Supervisor
The Johns Hopkins University Hospital
Baltimore, Maryland

Girolamo Sirchia, MD
Director, Blood Transfusion Service
Ospedale Policlinico
Milan, Italy

Special thanks are extended to Ortho Biotech for their generous support of the AABB's workshop, "Controversies in Transfusion Medicine: Immune Complications and Cytomegalovirus Transmission." We are grateful for their contribution to the success of this educational activity.

American Association of Blood Banks
Arlington, Virginia
1990

American Association of Blood Banks
1117 North 19th Street, Suite 600
Arlington, Virginia 22209

ISBN NO. 0-915355-87-6
First Printing
Printed in the United States

Library of Congress Cataloging-in-Publication Data

Controversies in transfusion medicine: immune complications and cytomegalovirus transmission/editors, Sanford R. Kurtz, Michael L. Baldwin, Girolamo Sirchia.
p. cm.
Includes bibliographical references.
Includes index.
ISBN 0-915355-87-6
1. Blood—Transfusion—Complications and sequelae—Prevention.
2. Blood—Effect of radiation on. 3. Cytomegalovirus infections—Prevention.
4. Graft versus host disease—Prevention. 5. Leucocyte-depleted blood products—Therapeutic use. I. Kurtz, Stanford R., 1947-
II. Baldwin, Michael L. III. Sirchia, Girolamo.
[DNLM: 1. Blood Component Removal. 2. Blood Transfusion—adverse effects. 3. Cytomegalic Inclusion Disease—transmission. 4. Graft vs Host Disease—Prevention & control. 5. Leukemia—therapy. WB 356 C764]
RM171.C586 1990
615'.39—dc20
DNLM/DLC
for Library of Congress
90-724
CIP

Technical/Scientific Workshops Committee

Dennis M. Smith, Jr., MD, Chairman

Michael L. Baldwin, MBA, MT(ASCP)SBB
Alice Reynolds Barr, SBB(ASCP)
Daniel B. Brubaker, DO
Katherine B. Carlson, MT(ASCP)SBB
Morris R. Dixon, MM, MT(ASCP)SBB
Ronnie J. Garner, MD
Frances L. Gibbs, MS, MT(ASCP)SBB
Avrum H. Golub, MD
Christina A. Kasprisin, MS, RN
Sanford R. Kurtz, MD
Barbara Laird-Fryer, MT(ASCP)SBB
Judith S. Levitt, MT(ASCP)SBB
Leo J. McCarthy, MD
JoAnn M. Moulds, MS, MT(ASCP)SBB
Ronald A. Sacher, MD
Stephanie Summers, PhD, MT(ASCP)SBB
Phyllis Unger, MT(ASCP)SBB
Margaret E. Wallace, MHS, MT(ASCP)SBB
Robert G. Westphal, MD
Susan M. Wilson, MT(ASCP)SBB

Contents

Foreword.. ix

1. **Leukocyte-Depleted Red Blood Cells for Transfusion.... 1**

   Girolamo Sirchia, MD; Anna Parravicini, ScD;
   Paolo Rebulla, MD; and Francesco Bertolini, MD

   Technical Considerations.. 3
   Clinical Experience 5
   References 7

2. **Leukocyte-Depleted Blood Components for Patients**
   With Leukemia or Aplastic Anemia—CON............... 13

   Kuo-Jang Kao, MD, PhD and Marsha F. Bertholf, MD

   Leukocyte-Poor vs Leukocyte-Depleted
      Blood Components 14
   Quantitative and Qualitative Significance of Donor
      Leukocytes... 15
   Routine Use of Leukocyte-Depleted Blood
      Components: Necessity or Extravagance?................... 22
   Conclusions and Recommendations 26
   References 27

3. **Leukocyte-Depleted Blood Components for Patients**
   With Leukemia or Aplastic Anemia—PRO 33

   Marlene M. Fisher, MB, BCh

   Leukocyte Mass in Absolute and Relative Terms 34
   Leukocyte-Poor Blood Components—Potential for
      Clinical Benefit... 35
   Methods for Leukocyte Depletion of Blood Components .. 44
   Immunomodulation by UV Irradiation 47
   Conclusions and Recommendations 48
   References 49

4. **Irradiation of Blood Components To Prevent**
   Graft-vs-Host Disease 57

   Kenneth C. Anderson, MD and Howard J. Weinstein, MD

   Historical Perspective 58

Who Is at Risk? 61
Factors Predisposing to GVHD-PT.................................. 66
Strategies for Prevention of Graft-vs-Host Disease
  Posttransfusion... 67
Conclusion and Recommendations 70
References.. 72

5. Cytomegalovirus Infection in Clinical Transplantation: The Role of Transfusion Support Using Donors Seronegative for Cytomegalovirus 81

Hayden G. Braine, MD

Molecular Biology of the Cytomegalovirus...................... 82
Spectrum of Disease Caused by CMV 84
Epidemiology of CMV Infection 86
Patterns of Infection Following Organ Transplantation ... 87
Approaches to Prevention of Posttransfusion
  CMV Infection 95
References.. 99

6. Cytomegalovirus-Seronegative Blood Support for Perinatal Patients—CON 103

Jutta K. Preiksaitis, MD

The Problem—A Historical Perspective 104
CMV and the Leukocyte... 107
Donor Factors That Influence the Risk of
  Transfusion-Acquired CMV Infection......................... 110
Recipient Factors That Influence the Risk of
  Transfusion-Acquired CMV Infection......................... 111
A Model for the Pathogenesis of Transfusion-Acquired
  CMV Infection 112
What Can We Learn From the Incidence of
  Transfusion-Acquired CMV Infection in
  Other Patient Populations?.. 113
How Can We Explain the Geographic Variability in
  Risk of Transfusion-Acquired CMV Infections
  in Neonatal Populations?... 115
Which Neonates Should Receive CMV-"Safe"
  Blood Components? 117
Alternatives to the Use of Seronegative Cellular Blood
  Components.. 120
References.. 123

7. **Cytomegalovirus-Seronegative Blood Support for Perinatal Patients—PRO** **131**

Nancy L. Dock, PhD

Characteristics of CMV 131
Neonatal Infection and Transfusion Studies 133
CMV Infection in the Donor 139
Means for Prevention 142
Blood Components and Treatments 144
Rationale for CMV-Negative Blood Support 145
Summary 148
References 149

Index **155**

Foreword

On first review this book seems to bring together three unrelated topics: leukocyte-depleted blood components for patients with leukemia and aplastic anemia, blood irradiation to prevent transfusion-induced graft-vs-host disease (GVHD) and cytomegalovirus (CMV)-negative blood support for pediatric and adult patients undergoing transplantation. However, these topics do have much in common. Clearly, they collectively represent some of the most difficult and contemporary issues involving transfusion medicine today. In addition, they all reinforce the important immunologic consequences of blood transfusion. Scientifically, they are all related to the presence of contaminating leukocytes in the blood products used to support patients. Finally, they all discuss how leukocyte removal or inactivation is beneficial to avoid morbidity and mortality from associated complications.

Improved understanding of blood cell physiology has stimulated major technological advances. Over the last 40 years this technology has driven improvements in transfusion-related patient care more than in any other time period. It has also permitted investigators to probe deeper into the mechanisms of viral diseases and the immunobiology of allogeneic blood transfusion. Although the pathophysiology of GVHD is not completely understood, we know that T lymphocytes play an important role. The DNA genome of CMV has been shown to be present in cells of the granulocyte and monocyte lineage as well as the T cell. The importance of monocytes, dendritic cells and lymphocytes in the development of alloimmunization following the transfusion of red cells and platelets is well established.

New technology (specifically, radiation treatment of blood components and the introduction of filters capable of improved removal of leukocytes by several logs) has also created problems. How should this technology be used? How should it be monitored? What quality control is required? Do the additional benefits offset the increased costs? The authors attempt to answer these questions for various clinical settings.

Leukocyte-depleted blood components and CMV-negative blood support for perinatal patients were presented in the workshop in a point/counterpoint manner with two authors taking opposing views on the same statement. An effort has been made to avoid duplication of information in this text.

Based on small-scale clinical studies, leukocyte-depleted blood component support in patients appears capable of preventing HLA alloimmunization. However, routine use seems premature at this time despite its importance for patients who are considered for unrelated allogeneic bone marrow transplantation. Patients with evidence of previous alloimmunization should be excluded but defining this population serologically is not straightforward. Careful quality control on the residual number of leukocytes transfused must be performed to ensure that no more than 5×10^6 leukocytes are transfused each time. The filters themselves are expensive and the cost/benefit must be established in various clinical settings.

We do not know enough about CMV transmission to utilize the technology that will soon permit mechanical removal of enough leukocytes to minimize CMV transmission from blood products. A majority of donors are serologically positive for CMV exposure but only a few are capable of transmitting the infection through transfusion of their blood. Correspondingly, not all recipients develop CMV disease despite receiving infectious material through transfusion. The immunosuppressive effect of blood transfusion may play a role in this process as well. In addition the affect of CMV on the host immune system can have serious consequences in the bone marrow transplant patient.

Finally, the development of transfusion related GVHD in immunocompetent adults following the transfusion of cellular blood products from first degree relatives of the recipient serves to remind us all of the exquisitely sensitive and complex systems challenged by the transfusion process which we frequently take for granted.

Sanford R. Kurtz, MD
Michael L. Baldwin, MBA, MT(ASCP)SBB
Girolamo Sirchia, MD
Editors

In: Kurtz SR, Baldwin ML and Sirchia G, eds.
Controversies in Transfusion Medicine:
Immune Complications and Cytomegalovirus Transmission
Arlington, VA: American Association
of Blood Banks,1990

1

Leukocyte-Depleted Red Blood Cells for Transfusion

Girolamo Sirchia, MD; Anna Parravicini, ScD;
Paolo Rebulla, MD; and Francesco Bertolini, MD

THE SAFETY OF BLOOD transfusion therapy increases if red blood cell (RBC) and platelet concentrates are depleted of their leukocyte content. This statement is supported by a number of facts. Foreign leukocytes can stimulate the production of alloantibodies directed against both HLA- and leukocyte-specific antigens in a large proportion of patients[1-3] who may thus develop nonhemolytic febrile transfusion reactions (NHFTR),[4,5] refractoriness to platelet transfusion[6,7] and rejection of organ or tissue transplants.[8] In paroxysmal nocturnal hemoglobinuria (PNH), a hemolytic anemia due to a red cell membrane abnormality that makes the cell highly susceptible to the lytic action of complement,[9] transfused leukocytes are a frequent cause of hemolytic transfusion reaction. In fact, by reacting with lymphocytotoxic antibodies, they activate complement in the fluid phase, causing lysis of PNH red cells by a mechanism of "reactive lysis."[10]

Transfusion of homologous leukocytes can also determine graft-vs-host disease (GVHD). This occurs more often in recipients with decreased immune defenses[11,12] (such as congenitally immunodeficient subjects, premature infants, patients infected with human immunodeficiency virus [HIV] and patients treated with aggressive chemo- or radiotherapy). How-

Girolamo Sirchia, MD, Director; Anna Parravicini, ScD, Technical Director; Paolo Rebulla, MD, Senior Assistant; Francesco Bertolini, MD, Assistant; Centro Trasfusionale e di Immunologia dei Trapianti, Ospedale Maggiore Policlinico, Milan, Italy

ever, it has recently been observed in fully immunocompetent surgical patients.[13-15] In the latter, GVHD could have been caused when fresh blood from a donor homozygous for a particular tissue antigen was transfused to a patient heterozygous for that antigen; the recipient did not recognize foreign leukocytes, whereas these latter recognized and reacted against the host's tissues. Foreign leukocytes are also the main vehicle of some lymphotropic viruses such as cytomegalovirus (CMV),[16,17] human T-cell lymphotropic virus type 1 (HTLV-I)[18] and Epstein-Barr virus (EBV).[19]

Lastly, homologous leukocytes are one, if not the most, important cause of the transfusion-induced immunosuppression observed in some pathological conditions. The best known example is the so-called "transfusion effect" exploited for years to improve kidney graft survival. The graft outcome is significantly better in patients who receive blood transfusions before transplantation than in patients who have never been transfused.[20] This is especially true in patients treated with a conventional immunosuppressive treatment (mainly azathioprine and corticosteroids) and is much less evident in the present era of cyclosporine therapy.[21]

That blood transfusion is capable of determining immunosuppression in some conditions is also apparent by the reactivation of endogenous CMV infections even in patients transfused with anti-CMV-negative blood,[22] by the increased postoperative infectious complications occurring in transfused

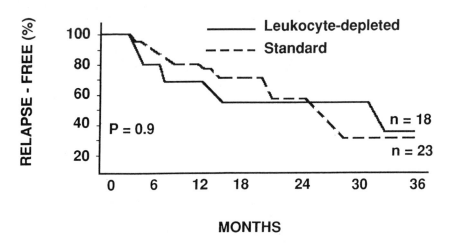

Figure 1-1. Analysis of duration of first remission in acute leukemia patients transfused with leukocyte-poor or standard blood components.[29]

surgical patients[23] and by reduced recurrences in Crohn's disease.[24] Moreover, even if more data are needed to reach a firm conclusion,[25] there is some evidence that frequency of tumor recurrences and mortality rates are increased in some types of tumor patients if they are transfused at surgery.[26,27] At variance with these observations is the finding of Tucker et al[28] who reported that in a small group of acute myeloblastic leukemia patients, the duration of remission appeared significantly shorter in recipients of leukocyte-depleted RBC and platelet concentrates compared to recipients of standard blood components, suggesting that transfused leukocytes may have a graft-vs-leukemia effect. However, the results of an Italian cooperative study that followed 41 acute leukemia patients do not support this conclusion (Fig 1-1).[29]

Technical Considerations

All in all, the above data indicate that leukocyte depletion of RBC (and platelet) concentrates is warranted. Until recently, leukocyte depletion of RBCs was carried out with the almost single purpose of preventing NHFTR. This is understandable not only because most knowledge of the harmful effect of transfused leukocytes is quite new, but also because the techniques for leukocyte depletion were cumbersome, difficult to standardize and often expensive.[30,31] They included differential centrifugation, sedimentation, washing, freezing and thawing.

The real breakthrough came when Diepenhorst et al prepared a filter that was capable of retaining at least 98% leukocytes, allowing a 96% red cell recovery.[32,33] By the mid-1970's, this filter (Erypur®, Organon Teknika, Oss, The Netherlands) was available on the market in Europe. A few years later a cotton-wool filter (Imugard IG500®, Terumo, Tokyo, Japan) was produced in Japan.[34] This filter also provided excellent leukocyte depletion and red cell recovery.

Most of these and subsequent leukocyte-depletion procedures were tested in our laboratory.[35] In addition, we had the opportunity of comparing most of them in a cohort of 80 transfusion-dependent homozygous thalassemia patients who have been followed for 10 years or more at our Department of Pediatrics and who receive periodic blood transfusions (10-15 mL of 1- to 7-day-old RBCs/kg body weight at 3-4 week intervals). For all the procedures of leukocyte depletion used over the years in these patients, the transfusion reaction rate and the patient reaction rate are available in addition to some other clinical information. In vitro each procedure evaluation includes red cell recovery and the number of residual leukocytes. Due to the inaccuracy of leukocyte counts by machine,[36] these are carried out manually in a Burker chamber, counting the number of leukocytes in 1.8 µL of a 1:10 suspension of blood in 2% acetic acid colored pale violet with gentian violet.[37]

In many laboratories, including our own, all the other methods were abandoned when Erypur® and Imugard IG500® became available. Moreover, in 1983 we found that Imugard IG500® worked very well also for leukocyte depletion of platelet concentrates,[38] a result later confirmed by other investigators.[39,40]

The advantages of leukocyte depletion by filtration, however, reached a peak when filtration at the bedside was introduced by Wenz et al.[41] These authors used Ultipor SQ40S® (Pall Corporation, Glen Cove, NY), a filter not specifically developed to retain leukocytes but microaggregates. They showed that if a unit of RBCs is spun at high speed and transfused to the patient through this filter, most NHFTRs could be prevented since the filter retains 71-83% of the leukocytes,[42,43] including most of the granulocytes, which are known to be the major factor responsible for the febrile reaction.[44] The advantages of this bedside filtration (called spin and filter) were the reduced workload compared with other leukocyte removal procedures and its low cost. Moreover, it was carried out in a closed system and caused no delay in providing leukocyte-depleted RBCs and no blood wastage if transfusion was cancelled.

After the experience of Wenz and coworkers, many filters suitable for use at the bedside were produced by different companies. Three types of bedside filters have been adopted in our hospital to provide leukocyte-depleted RBCs: Pall SQ40S®, Sepacell R500® (Asahi, Tokyo, Japan) and Pall RC100®. Pall SQ40S® was used in 1985 in the spin, cool and filter procedure,[43] a modification of spin and filter. According to this procedure, RBCs were spun at high speed and refrigerated for at least 3 hours at 4 C before filtration to increase the coalescence of microaggregates. This procedure showed the advantage of high red cell recovery, leukocyte depletion of 82-92% (Table 1-1)[43] and an acceptable transfusion rate when 50 mL saline were infused in the transfusion set, with the disadvantages of the need for precentrifugation and careful handling of the bag.

From November 1985 to September 1988 our patients received RBCs filtered at the bedside through Sepacell R500®.[45] This filter was found effective in removing leukocytes but with

Table 1-1. Effectiveness of Different Bedside Filters Used in Milan

Filter Type	RBC Units per Filter (no.)	Red Cell Recovery (%)	Residual Leukocytes (x10^6)	In Vivo Infusion Time/Unit (min)
Ultipor SQ40S® (n = 40)	1	93* (82-98)†	360 (110-1100)	65 (55-105)
Sepacell R500® (n = 26)	1	63 (53-79)	0 (0-2)	65 (30->150)
	2	82 (75-89)	0 (0-24)	
Pall RC100® (n = 80)	1	90 (73-99)	0 (0-32)	35 (25-65)
	2	93 (84-100)	9 (0-195)	

*Median
†Range

standard RBCs it showed a slow and variable infusion rate and a low red cell recovery, which became even lower when the volume of the filter was increased to improve blood flow and leukocyte removal.

Pall RC100® became available in October 1988. The results obtained with this filter are reported in Table 1-1. Pall RC100® has given very satisfactory results in terms of red cell recovery, leukocyte removal, infusion rate and simplicity of use.[46]

Clinical Experience

Figure 1-2 summarizes the clinical experience in our setting with the main procedures of leukocyte depletion used to transfuse our thalassemia patients in the past decade. It appears that the increased effectiveness of the procedures used for preparing leukocyte-depleted RBCs was paralleled by a reduction of both patient and transfusion reaction rates. While until the recent past the main goal of leukocyte depletion was to prevent NHFTRs in selected patients, the high effectiveness and ease of use of last generation bedside filters stimulate the achievement of the more ambitious goal of avoiding other important complications of blood transfusion as well.

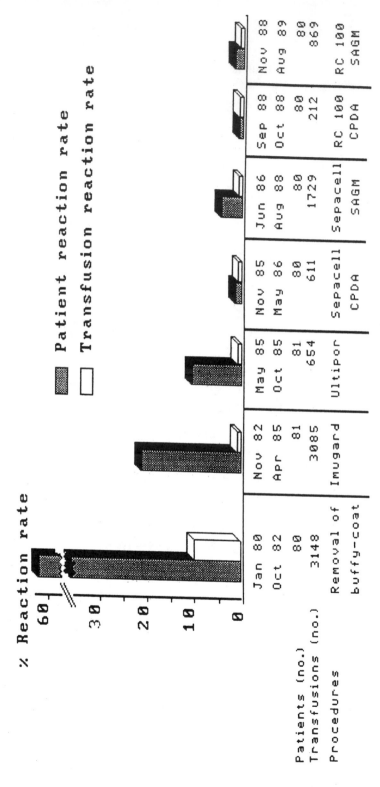

Figure 1-2. Transfusion and patient reaction rates in the group of thalassemics transfused at our hospital since 1980 with red blood cells depleted of leukocytes with different methods.

The time has probably come when the use of RBCs depleted of leukocytes by procedures that allow 3-4 log removal rates becomes routine for patients who are chronically transfused, immunosuppressed (newborn, transplanted, cancer and HIV-infected patients) and candidates for transplantation. It remains to be evaluated if this procedure should be used also for other categories of patients and eventually for all blood transfusion recipients. For this purpose, a cost/benefit analysis is needed.

Benefits include prevention of NHFTR, of antileukocyte antibody production in previously nonstimulated thalassemics[47] and in a proportion of leukemia patients[48-51] and of CMV transmission,[52-54] which have already been demonstrated. Prevention of GVHD in immunosuppressed and nonimmunosuppressed patients and of HTLV-I transmission seems possible. Prevention of immunosuppression in some conditions (like cancer) and of transmission of viruses integrated into the donor's genome requires further investigation.

Present costs preclude the use of filtered blood components for all recipients of blood transfusion; however, the cost of the product depends on the number of pieces produced and could be much lower than it is now if some million filters per year were produced. Moreover, it is conceivable that in the future new more economic technologies will be developed. In addition, reduction of some present costs, such as those connected with screening blood donors for anti-CMV, managing a group of HLA-typed blood donors for the treatment of platelet refractoriness, cost of the liability of transfusion complications and cost of management of immunized patients waiting for organ transplantation, should also be considered. When this economic analysis is performed, the use of leukocyte-depleted blood components could become routine.

References

1. Barton JC. Nonhemolytic, noninfectious transfusion reactions. Semin Hematol 1981;18:95-121.
2. Décary F, Ferner P, Giavedoni L, et al. An investigation of nonhemolytic transfusion reactions. Vox Sang 1984;46: 277-85.
3. De Rie MA, Plas-van Dalen CM van der, Engelfriet CP, Borne AEG Kr von dem. The serology of febrile transfusion reactions. Vox Sang 1985;49:126-34.

4. Payne R. The association of febrile transfusion reactions with leuko-agglutinins. Vox Sang 1957;2:233-41.
5. Brittingham TE, Chaplin H Jr. Febrile transfusion reactions caused by sensitivity to donor leukocytes and platelets. JAMA 1957;165:819-25.
6. Herzig RH, Herzig GP, Bull MI, et al. Correction of poor platelet transfusion responses with leukocyte-poor HLA-matched platelet concentrates. Blood 1975;46:743-50.
7. Eernisse JG, Brand A. Prevention of platelet refractoriness due to HLA antibodies by administration of leukocyte-poor blood components. Exp Hematol 1981;9:77-83.
8. Kissmeyer-Nielsen F, Olsen S, Petersen Posborg V, Fjeldborg O. Hyperacute rejection of kidney allografts associated with pre-existing humoral antibodies against donor cells. Lancet 1966;2:662-5.
9. Rosse WF. Transfusion in paroxysmal nocturnal hemoglobinuria. To wash or not to wash? Transfusion 1989;29:663-4.
10. Sirchia G, Ferrone S, Mercuriali F. Leukocyte antigen-antibody reaction and lysis of paroxysmal nocturnal hemoglobinuria erythrocytes. Blood 1970;36:334-6.
11. Hathaway WE, Fulginiti VA, Pierce CW, et al. Graft-versus-host reactions following a single blood transfusion. JAMA 1967;201:1015-20.
12. Ford JM, Lucey JJ, Cullen MH, et al. Fatal graft-versus-host disease following transfusion of granulocytes from normal donors. Lancet 1976;2:1167-9.
13. Juji T, Takahashi K, Shibata Y, et al. Post-transfusion graft-versus-host disease in immunocompetent patients after cardiac surgery in Japan. N Engl J Med 1989;321:56.
14. Thaler M, Shamiss A, Orgad S, et al. The role of blood from HLA-homozygous donors in fatal transfusion-associated graft-versus-host disease after open-heart surgery. N Engl J Med 1989;321:25-8.
15. Otsuka S, Kunieda K, Hirose M, et al. Fatal erythroderma (suspected graft-versus-host disease) after cholecystectomy. Retrospective analysis. Transfusion 1989;29:544-8.
16. Rinaldo CR Jr, Black PH, Hirsh MS. Interaction of cytomegalovirus with leucocytes from patients with mononucleosis due to cytomegalovirus. J Infect Dis 1977; 136:667-78.
17. Schrier RD, Nelson JA, Oldstone MBA. Detection of human cytomegalovirus in peripheral blood lymphocytes in a natural infection. Science 1985;230:1048-51.

18. Okochi K, Sato H, Hinuma Y. A retrospective study on transmission of adult T-cell leukemia virus by blood transfusion: Seroconversion in recipients. Vox Sang 1984;46: 245-53.
19. Tolkoff-Rubin NE, Rubin RH, Keller EE, et al. Cytomegalovirus infection in dialysis patients and personnel. Ann Intern Med 1978;89:625-8.
20. Opelz G, Sengar DPS, Mickey MR, Terasaki PI. Effect of blood transfusions on subsequent kidney transplants. Transplant Proc 1973;5:253-9.
21. Opelz G for the Collaborative Transplant Study. Comparison of the transfusion effect in North America and Europe. Transplant Proc 1988;20:1069-70.
22. Adler SP, Baggett J, McVoy M. Transfusion-associated cytomegalovirus infections in seropositive cardiac surgery patients. Lancet 1985;2:743-6.
23. Tartter PI. Blood transfusion and postoperative infections. Transfusion 1989;29:456-9.
24. Williams JG, Hughes LE. Effect of perioperative blood transfusion on recurrence of Crohn's disease. Lancet 1989; 2:131-3.
25. Tartter PI, Francis DMA. Blood transfusion and tumor growth. Transplant Proc 1988;20:1108-11.
26. Foster RS Jr, Costanza M, Foster JC, et al. Blood transfusions and survival after resection of cancers of the breast, colon and lung: The need for prospective randomized trials. Transplant Proc 1988;20:1125-7.
27. Blumberg N, Heal JM. Transfusion and host defenses against cancer recurrence and infection. Transfusion 1989;29:236-45.
28. Tucker J, Murphy MF, Gregory WM, et al. Apparent removal of graft-versus-leukaemia effect by the use of leucocyte-poor blood components in patients with acute myeloblastic leukaemia. Br J Haematol 1989;73:572-81.
29. Rebulla P, Pappalettera M, Barbui T, et al. Duration of first remission in leukaemic recipients of leucocyte-poor blood components (letter). Br J Haematol 1990;75:441-2.
30. Wenz B. Leukocyte-free red cells: The evolution of a safer blood product. In: McCarthy LJ, Baldwin ML, eds. Controversies of leukocyte-poor blood and components. Arlington, VA: American Association of Blood Banks, 1989: 27-48.
31. Sirchia G, Parravicini A, Rebulla P. Leucocyte-depleted blood components. In: Cash JD, ed. Progress in transfu-

sion medicine. Edinburgh: Churchill Livingstone, 1988; 3:87-109.

32. Diepenhorst P, Sprokholt R, Prins HK. Removal of leukocytes from whole blood and erythrocyte suspensions by filtration through cotton wool. I. Filtration technique. Vox Sang 1972;23:308-20.

33. Diepenhorst P, Engelfriet CP. Removal of leukocytes from whole blood and erythrocyte suspensions by filtration through cotton wool. V. Results after transfusion of 1820 units of filtered erythrocytes. Vox Sang 1975;29:15-22.

34. Kikugawa K, Minoshima K. Filter columns for preparation of leukocyte-poor blood for transfusion. Vox Sang 1978; 34:281-90.

35. Sirchia G, Parravicini A, Rebulla P, et al. Evaluation of three procedures for the preparation of leukocyte-poor and leukocyte-free red blood cells for transfusion. Vox Sang 1980;38:197-204.

36. Milner GR, Fagence R, Darnborough J. Temperature dependence of leukocyte depletion of blood with an automatic blood cell processor. Transfusion 1982;22:48-50.

37. Dacie JV, Lewis SM. Practical haematology, 5th ed. Edinburgh: Churchill Livingstone, 1975.

38. Sirchia G, Parravicini A, Rebulla P, et al. Preparation of leukocyte-free platelets for transfusion by filtration through cotton wool. Vox Sang 1983;44:115-20.

39. Sniecinski I, St. Jean J, Nowicki B. Preparation of leukocyte-poor platelets by filtration. J Clin Apheresis 1989; 5:7-11.

40. Holme S, Ross D, Heaton WA. In vitro and in vivo evaluation of platelet concentrates after cotton wool filtration. Vox Sang 1989;57:112-5.

41. Wenz B, Gurtlinger KF, O'Toole AM, Dugan EP. Preparation of granulocyte-poor red blood cells by microaggregate filtration. A simplified method to minimize febrile transfusion reactions. Vox Sang 1980;39:282-7.

42. Wenz B. Microaggregate blood filtration and the febrile transfusion reaction. A comparative study. Transfusion 1983;23:95-8.

43. Parravicini A, Rebulla P, Apuzzo J, et al. The preparation of leukocyte-poor red cells for transfusion by a simple cost-effective technique. Transfusion 1984;24:508-9.

44. Perkins HA, Payne R, Ferguson J, Wood M. Nonhemolytic febrile transfusion reactions. Quantitative effects of blood components with emphasis on isoantigenic incompatibility of leukocytes. Vox Sang 1966;11:578-600.

45. Sirchia G, Rebulla P, Parravicini A, et al. Leukocyte depletion of red cell units at the bedside by transfusion through a new filter. Transfusion 1987;27:402-5.
46. Sirchia G, Wenz B, Rebulla P, et al. Removal of white cells from red cells by transfusion through a new filter. Transfusion 1990;30:30-3.
47. Sirchia G, Rebulla P, Mascaretti L, et al. The clinical importance of leukocyte depletion in regular erythrocyte transfusions. Vox Sang 1986;51(Suppl 1):2-8.
48. Murphy MF, Metcalfe P, Thomas H, et al. Use of leukocyte-poor blood components and HLA-matched-platelet donors to prevent HLA alloimmunization. Br J Haematol 1986;62: 529-34.
49. Sniecinski I, O'Donnell MR, Nowicki B, Hill LR. Prevention of refractoriness and HLA-alloimmunization using filtered blood products. Blood 1988;71:1402-7.
50. Andreu G, Dewailly J, Leberre C, et al. Prevention of HLA immunization with leukocyte-poor packed red cells and platelet concentrates obtained by filtration. Blood 1988; 72:964-9.
51. Brand A, Claas FHJ, Voogt RJ, et al. Alloimmunization after leukocyte-depleted multiple random donor platelet transfusions. Vox Sang 1988;54:160-6.
52. Gilbert GL, Hayes K, Hudson IL, James J, and the Neonatal Cytomegalovirus Infection Study Group. Prevention of transfusion-acquired cytomegalovirus infection in infants by blood filtration to remove leucocytes. Lancet 1989;1: 1228-31.
53. Murphy MF, Grint PCA, Hardiman AE, et al. Use of leucocyte-poor blood components to prevent primary cytomegalovirus (CMV) infection in patients with acute leukaemia. Br J Haematol 1988;70:253-5.
54. De Graan-Hentzen YCE, Gratama JW, Mudde GC, et al. Prevention of primary cytomegalovirus infection in patients with hematologic malignancies by intensive white cell depletion of blood products. Transfusion 1989;29: 757-60.

In: Kurtz SR, Baldwin ML and Sirchia G, eds.
Controversies in Transfusion Medicine:
Immune Complications and Cytomegalovirus Transmission
Arlington, VA: American Association
of Blood Banks, 1990

2

Leukocyte-Depleted Blood Components for Patients With Leukemia or Aplastic Anemia—CON

Kuo-Jang Kao, MD, PhD and Marsha F. Bertholf, MD

D URING THE 1980's, RAPID advances were made in the treatment of aplastic anemia and malignancies of both hematologic and solid tissues. More potent chemotherapeutic regimens and broader indications for bone marrow transplantation have been introduced and have created a need for more intensive blood component support. Consequently, this compromised patient population challenges transfusion services to provide specialized blood components in order to reduce the risks of cytomegalovirus (CMV) infection, human leukocyte antigen (HLA), alloimmunization, platelet transfusion refractoriness, graft-vs-host disease (GVHD) and recurrent nonhemolytic febrile transfusion reactions (NHFTR). All of these complications have been attributed to the presence of leukocytes in blood and blood components.

CMV infection, GVHD and febrile reactions can be effectively prevented by donor testing, by irradiation and by washing or filtering, respectively, to remove leukocytes from blood components. However, the effectiveness of using leukocyte-poor blood

Kuo-Jang Kao, MD, PhD, Associate Professor of Pathology, University of Florida and Director, Blood Bank, Shands. Hospital and Marsha F. Bertholf, MD, Instructor of Pathology, University of Florida, Gainesville, Florida. (This work was supported by a grant from the National Institutes of Health.)

and blood components to reduce HLA alloimmunization and prevent consequent platelet transfusion refractoriness has been limited. The inconsistent and insufficient leukocyte removal may be one contributing factor. Thus, great emphasis has been placed on the development of more effective and reliable techniques to deplete or inactivate leukocytes in blood components prior to transfusion. Filters highly efficient at removing leukocytes from blood components have become available recently. This technological advancement ushers transfusion services into the era of leukocyte-depleted blood components. Various potential benefits are being promised but with a higher price tag.

This chapter will review the mechanism by which donor leukocytes alloimmunize recipients against HLA antigens and examine the effectiveness of routine use of leukocyte-depleted blood components to prevent HLA alloimmunization. Other potential uses of leukocyte-depleted blood and blood components are also discussed.

Leukocyte-Poor vs Leukocyte-Depleted Blood Components

Recent technological progress has led to the availability of new third-generation filters for easy depletion of leukocytes from blood components by 2 to 3 logs (99-99.9%).[1-3] In comparison to filters such as Sepacell R-500® (Asahi, Tokyo, Japan), Imugard IG500® (Terumo, Tokyo, Japan) and Ultipor SQ40S® (Pall Corporation, Glen Cove, NY), the newly developed filters offer a 10-fold improvement in the efficiency of leukocyte removal. Similar progress is being made to introduce improved apheresis ma-chines able to prepare single donor platelet concentrates that contain equally low numbers of leukocytes.

All of these exciting developments finally allow scientific investigation of the potential use of leukocyte-depleted blood to prevent HLA alloimmunization. Nevertheless, the collection of data to answer this question has yet to be completed. Thus, the less expensive second generation or earlier version of third generation filters will continue to play a major role in transfusion medicine, and a distinction between blood components with different degrees of leukocyte removal becomes necessary. One suggestion is the use of "leukocyte-poor blood components" for those units containing $>5 \times 10^6$ residual leukocytes and "leukocyte-depleted blood components" for those containing $\leq 5 \times 10^6$ leukocytes. This distinction is made because most blood components will contain less than 5×10^6 leukocytes after filtration through the newly developed high efficiency filters and 5×10^6 leukocytes per transfusion may be the threshold dose necessary to reduce the risk of HLA alloimmunization.

Quantitative and Qualitative Significance of Donor Leukocytes

Leukocytes in Blood Components

Leukocytes are inherent contaminants in both packed red cells and platelet concentrates because the density of leukocytes is intermediate to that of red cells and platelets. On average, there are 3.2×10^9 leukocytes in a unit of unmodified whole blood[4] and most remain with packed red cells during preparation of various blood components. When 20 units of packed red blood cells (PRBCs) from our local blood center with ≤14 days of in vitro storage were randomly selected for quantitation of leukocytes, the average number per unit was $2.35 \pm 0.78 \times 10^9$ (mean ± SD) with a range of 0.99 to 4.05×10^9 white cells. The average differential counts for lymphocytes, monocytes and granulocytes as determined by Coulter S plus IV (Coulter Electronics, Hialeah, FL) in those 20 units were 49.6 ± 8.7%, 28.4 ± 7.4% and 22.0 ± 10.4%, respectively.

Numbers of contaminating leukocytes in random donor platelet concentrates (RDP) vary significantly according to centrifugation condition and harvesting technique.[5,6] The degree of contamination, therefore, is widely variable among blood centers. Reported average leukocyte counts per unit of RDPs range from 4.2×10^7 to 8.4×10^8 cells.[5-9] Most commonly, there are 7.0-9.0×10^7 leukocytes per unit of RDP.[5-9] Differential leukocyte counts performed on 10 units of RDPs obtained from our local blood center revealed 88.8 ± 4.8% lymphocytes, 7.2 ± 3.7% monocytes and 4.1 ± 1.9% granulocytes.

The degree of leukocyte contamination in single donor platelet concentrates (SDP) is also technique- and donor-dependent.[10] The numbers of leukocytes in SDPs obtained from our local blood center vary widely ranging from 0.5 to 20×10^8 (n=11). The average white cell load for a unit of SDPs is 5.6 ± 5.9×10^8 cells.

Functionally, most polymorphonuclear granulocytes in red cell units begin to lose bactericidal activity 24 hours after blood collection and have no significantly detectable bactericidal activity 4 days later under standard blood bank storage at 4 C.[11] This loss of function coincides with increased numbers of cells with degenerative morphological changes.[11] In contrast, 30% of lymphocytes still maintain their normal morphology after 21 days of storage at 4 C.[11] Incorporation of tritiated thymidine by lymphocytes following stimulation of phytohemagglutinin (PHA) does not change until 10 days after blood collection.[11] At our institution, more than 90% of PRBCs are transfused within 10 days after collection. Thus, a significant number of functional lymphocytes and occasion-ally viable granulocytes are infused into recipients along with red cells.

Recent studies demonstrate that more than 90% of leukocytes in RDP concentrates remain viable after storage for 5 days and there is no significant change in the ability of mononuclear cells to respond to PHA stimulation or to function as respon-ders in mixed leukocyte culture (MLC) reaction.[7,8] Nevertheless, a 70% reduction in the ability to be stimulator cells in MLC is observed following 5 days' storage.[8] This decline most likely is related to a selective loss of nonlymphoid monocytes or dendritic cells, because they are the cells primarily responsible for stimulator function in MLC.[12]

Variables such as the number of cells, the cell types and the viability of leukocytes can be important attributes for determining the alloantigenicity of each blood component and may have a significant clinical importance.

Quantitative Distribution of HLA Antigen in Blood

Class I HLA antigens are polymorphic membrane glycoproteins that are expressed on the surface of most nucleated cells[12] and platelets,[13,14] and are also present in plasma.[14,15] These molecules exist as heterodimers that consist of a 44-kD heavy chain and a noncovalently associated 12-kD β_2-microglobulin.[16] HLA antigens play important roles in the presentation of antigenic peptides to cytotoxic T lymphocytes.[17] They are also the major target for antibodies and cytotoxic T lymphocytes during graft rejection.[16] As reported earlier,[18] the distribution of HLA antigens in different components of whole blood is approximately 67% on platelets, 27% in plasma, 2% on lymphocytes, 2% on granulocytes and 2% on red blood cells. Thus, platelets and plasma HLA account for more than 90% of total HLA antigens in whole blood. Using the reported HLA concentrations[18] for platelets, red cells and plasma to calculate the amount of HLA antigens in a unit of PRBCs with 0.80 (80%) hematocrit, there is 90 µg of HLA antigens in a unit of PRBC with 50% of the antigens present on red cells. In a unit of RDPs, there is 800 µg of HLA with 90% present on platelets. Because patients with acute leukemia or aplastic anemia are often platelet transfusion dependent and allogeneic bone marrow transplantation is one therapeutic option for them, it is clinically important to prevent HLA alloimmunization in these patients. Since significant amounts of HLA antigens are present in all different components of blood, patients with leukemia or aplastic anemia inevitably will be frequently challenged with high doses of foreign HLA antigens through blood transfusions regardless of how completely leukocytes are depleted from blood components.

Class II molecules of the major histocompatibility complex (MHC) such as DP, DQ and DR antigens are also integral membrane proteins and consist of two noncovalently associated polypeptide chains.[19,20] These antigens are present on B lymphocytes and monocytes/dendritic cells in peripheral blood.[19,20] Functionally, they are pivotal in presenting antigenic peptides to helper T lymphocytes.[20] Since Class II MHC antigens are present only on B lymphocytes and monocytes/dendritic cells, the total amount of Class II MHC in blood is much less than Class I HLA. It has been reported that only 6% of lymphocytes in RDP are positive for Class II MHC antigens.[8] Thus, it is expected that the amount of Class II MHC transfused through blood components is significantly less than Class I HLA. It is not clear whether the lower quantity of Class II MHC will have a lower antigenicity. Because Class II MHC antigens are not detectable on platelets,[21] the antibodies against Class II MHC therefore are not directly responsible for immunological refractoriness to platelet transfusions in multitransfused patients.

Mechanisms of HLA Alloimmunization

Although high concentrations of HLA antigens are present in PRBC and platelet concentrates, the often-reported incidence of alloimmunization against HLA after multiple transfusions in leukemic aplastic anemia patients is between 30 and 60%.[22-30] Therefore, a significant number of patients do not develop any anti-HLA antibodies, and may belong to the so-called "nonresponder" group. Furthermore, experimental work using highly purified platelets to induce primary alloimmunization against Class I molecules of MHC in mice,[31] mongrel dogs[32] and rhesus monkeys[33] indicates that Class I MHC antigens by themselves are not very immunogenic. Similar observations have also been made in humans.[34] These studies suggest that contaminating leukocytes in blood components may play a critical role in the induction of alloimmunization against HLA antigens.

This conclusion is substantiated by the study using long-term in vitro tissue culture of allografts to eliminate passenger leukocytes and to reduce their immunogenicity for successful engraftment.[35] A subsequent study further demon-strated that elimination of Ia antigen positive leukocytes also reduced the alloimmunogenicity of allografts.[36] More importantly, the same effects can be achieved by irradiating allograft or platelet concentrates with short wavelength UV light to inactivate contaminating leukocytes.[37,38] These findings indicate that certain subset(s) of metabolically active and Ia-positive passenger leukocytes in allografts may be responsible for alloimmunizing recipients and leading to graft rejection.

It has been shown that the pretreatment of mouse splenic or human peripheral blood leukocytes with 8-methoxypsoralene (8-MOP) and irradiation with long wave-length UV light (UV-A) effectively inactivates donor leukocytes as stimulator cells in mixed leukocyte culture.[39] By using the same treatment on mouse platelet concentrates, the alloantigenicity of Class I MHC is significantly reduced and more transfusions of 8-MOP and UV-A treated platelet concentrates are necessary to alloimmunize recipient mice.[40] The titers of antibodies against Class I MHC in mice receiving 8-MOP and UV-A treated platelets are also significantly lower. The pretreatment by 8-MOP and UV-A irradiation induces covalent crosslinkage of DNA and leads to inhibition of m-RNA transcription and cell proliferation.[41,42] Thus, the success of using 8-MOP and UV-A treatment to reduce Class I MHC alloantigenicity highly suggests that a certain co-stimulatory factor(s) from donor leukocyte is required to initiate immune response against foreign Class I MHC antigens in recipients and that the putative co-stimulatory factor(s) is not expressed constitutively and needs to be synthesized during the initial stage of allosensitization.

As reported previously, interleukin-1 (IL-1) secreted from antigen-presenting cells plays an important role in triggering immune response and IL-1 is not expressed in resting antigen-presenting cells until they are activated.[43] In addition, leukocytes with positive Ia or DR antigens only include monocytes, dendritic cells and B-lymphocytes.[44] It is also known that monocytes and dendritic cells are the major antigen-presenting cells.[44] Based on these findings, the sequence of events in primary HLA allosensitization may take place as follows (Fig 2-1).

Once viable and metabolically active monocytes and/or dendritic cells are transfused into a recipient, alloreactive helper T lymphocytes in recipients react with DR molecules on donor monocytes and/or dendritic cells through T-cell receptors.[45,46] This interaction leads to activation of monocytes and/or dendritic cells. The key interleukins, such as IL-1 and IL-6 are synthesized and secreted to initiate alloimmune response. Secreted or membrane-bound IL-1 stimulates recipient helper T lymphocytes to proliferate and to release IL-2 and other interleukins.[47] Concomitantly, IL-1 enhances B-cell response to antigen-specific or nonspecific T-cell help,[48-50] leading to eventual allosensitization with production of alloantibody against HLA antigens. However, it is not known whether alloreactive helper T lymphocytes of the recipient recognize bare donor DR molecules or DR molecules with bound self-HLA

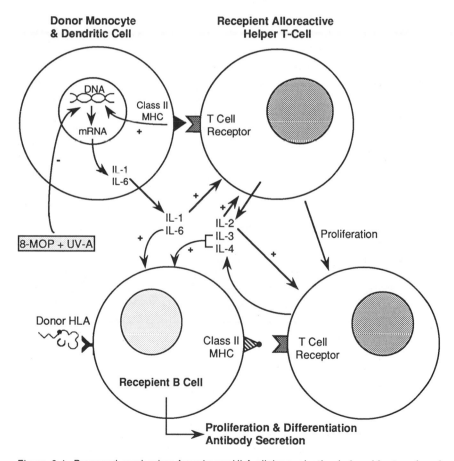

Figure 2-1. Proposed mechanism for primary HLA alloimmunization induced by transfused donor monocytes and dendritic cells. Pretreatment of platelet concentrates with 8-methoxypsoralen (8-MOP) and UV-A irradiation prevents the synthesis and subsequent release of interleukins IL-1 and IL-6. Consequently, immune response to donor Class I MHC antigens is inhibited. (= inhibition; + = activation.)

peptides from donors. It is also not yet clear whether T-cell receptor on the recipient's alloreactive T-helper lymphocytes cross-reacts with self DR molecules bound with foreign HLA peptides or not. All of these important questions need to be further studied. Recently, Lagaaij et al[51] reported that transfusions with one HLA-DR antigen-matched red cells significantly reduce the incidence of HLA alloimmunization in patients awaiting kidney or heart transplants. Their finding demonstrates the significance of DR disparity for interaction between the recipient alloreactive helper T cell and the donor leukocyte in initiation of HLA alloimmunization.

Previously, Pellegrino et al[52] reported that repeated infusions of HLA antigens in 50 mL of plasma were able to alloimmunize two out of seven chronic renal insufficiency patients who had no prior blood transfusion and/or pregnancy. Nonetheless, the cytotoxic antibodies could be detected only by using cultured lymphoid cell lines, not by peripheral blood lymphocytes. Since the cultured lymphoid cell lines express more HLA antigens than circulating lymphocytes, the results suggest that lower titers of anti-HLA antibodies were developed in those two individuals. Their studies indicate that plasma HLA antigens can be processed by antigen-presenting cells of recipients to initiate immune response through the classical pathway. Since more than 90% of HLA antigens in donor whole blood are present in plasma and on platelets,[18] removal of all leukocytes from donor blood components may only reduce the alloantigenicity of these blood components and cannot completely prevent primary alloimmunization against HLA antigens.

Studies in renal patients with prior HLA alloimmunization and subsequent loss of anti-HLA antibodies also show that the use of leukocyte-depleted red cell units cannot prevent the anamnestic response.[53,54] The HLA antibodies often re-emerged shortly after transfusions with only one or two units of leukocyte-depleted and washed red cells. The quantity of HLA antigens on red cells appears sufficient to trigger the anamnestic response.

Quantitative Importance of Transfused Donor Leukocytes

Based on the foregoing review, it becomes apparent that donor leukocytes, most likely monocytes and/or dendritic cells, are primarily responsible for HLA alloantigenicity in blood components and that the initial alloimmunization may be prevented or delayed by leukocyte depletion. An immediate concrn regarding the use of leukocyte-depleted blood components for prevention of alloimmunization is whether the quantity of donor leukocytes remaining in such a blood component will still be able to effectively cause the HLA alloantigenicity.

No study has been done to specifically measure the threshold dose of leukocytes necessary to provoke primary HLA alloimmunization. However, several previous studies have partially addressed the issue. Claas et al,[31] reported that at least 1×10^3 leukocytes in platelet concentrates are needed to allosen-sitize recipient mice, but 1×10^2 leukocytes were sufficient for an anamnestic antibody response. These doses correspond to 10^6 and 10^5 leukocytes, respectively, in man. Interestingly, these values are quite similar to what have been observed in human studies. Fisher et al,[26] reported that three biweekly transfusions of platelet suspensions containing as few as 1.5×10^7 leukocytes led to the development of alloantibody in 4 of 12 patients. None of 12 patients who received less than 5×10^6 leukocytes during each transfusion became allosensitized. The results suggest that the threshold immunogenic dose most likely is between 10^6 and 10^7 leukocytes. Although other studies[27,28,30] reported that the incidences of allosensitization can be significantly lowered with transfusions of blood containing residual white cells higher than 4.7×10^7, it would be prudent to infuse less than 5×10^6 leukocytes during each transfusion in order to avoid primary HLA alloimmunization based on available evidence.

Quality Control for Leukocyte-Depleted Blood Components

As mentioned earlier, there are a mean of 2.4×10^9 leukocytes in a unit of packed red cells and approximately 4.2×10^8 white cells in a pool of 6 units of RDPs. In order to obtain leukocyte counts less than 5×10^6, more than 99.8% and 98.8% of contaminating white cells need to be removed from packed red cells and pooled RDP, respectively. However, the reported efficiencies for leukocyte depletion from red cell units and pooled random donor platelets using the high efficiency filters were 97.5-99.8%[2,55-58] and 94-99.8%,[1,2,59,60] respectively. The actual performance may fall short of what has been promised by the manufacturers. In addition, it is not uncommon to have much higher starting concentrations of leukocytes in units of PRBCs or SDPs which can also contribute to insufficient depletion of leukocytes. Both factors emphasize the need for frequent quality control of high-efficiency filters in order to ensure that the filtered PRBCs or pooled RDPs indeed contain less than the immunogenic dose of leukocytes after filtration.

It is also important to establish the correctness of each new leukocyte depletion procedure by performing leukocyte counting on every unit of the first 10-20 units of blood components processed by the new procedure. Thereafter, intermittent biweekly or monthly quality control should be performed.

Simple and reliable methods for accurate quantitation of leukocytes at a concentration of $<5 \times 10^6$ cells per 300 mL, or 17 cells per μL, become necessary. Since automated counters are not adequate to quantify such a low concentration of leukocytes, the manual chamber count becomes the method of choice.[2] But since a dense background of cellular debris and unlysed red cells or platelets frequently interferes with enumeration of nucleated leukocytes, modification of the existing method of chamber count is needed. Among several recently reported methods for counting low numbers of leukocytes,[58,61,62] the use of fluorescence microscopy to identify and enumerate the nuclei of leukocytes stained with propidium iodide is the simplest. This method permits easy and reliable determination of leukocyte concentration as low as 1 cell/μL in filtered RDPs or 11 cells/μL in PRBCs.[61] The sensitivity is more than needed to detect 5×10^6 cells in filtered blood components. Moreover, the limit of detection can be further improved by counting cells in higher volumes of propidium iodide stained samples in hemacytometers.

Routine Use of Leukocyte-Depleted Blood Components: Necessity or Extravagance?

Although the growing availability of various high efficiency leukocyte-removal filters enables removal of contaminating leukocytes by 2 to 3 log, controversies as to the benefit of routine use of leukocyte-depleted blood components remain.

Prevention of HLA Alloimmunization

Since metabolically active donor leukocytes (most likely monocytes and dendritic cells) are essential to allosensitize recipients against HLA antigens, thorough depletion of leukocytes from blood components should prevent or delay the primary HLA alloimmunization. Nevertheless, the degree of leukocyte depletion that needs to be achieved in order to ensure the success of prevention of HLA alloimmunization is not known. The data available thus far are conflicting. The number of residual leukocytes that effectively reduced the incidence of alloimmunization in some studies failed to do so in others.[24-30] The small number of patients in many of those studies also precludes deriving any firm conclusion. Furthermore, the inclusion of patients with different diagnoses, chemotherapy regimens and histories of previous pregnancy and/or transfusion further complicates the analysis of data. More importantly, the endpoint measurement for alloimmunization was frequently defined as positive reaction against more than 10% or 20% of panel lymphocytes.[25,29,30] This definition of endpoint could falsely underestimate the incidence of alloimmunization in patients receiving leukocyte-depleted blood components.

Another area of major concern is the efficacy of using leukocyte-depleted blood components to prevent anamnestic response, especially in those previously alloimmunized patients with undetectable anti-HLA antibodies by lymphocytotoxicity tests.[63] As discussed earlier, HLA antigens on red blood cells may be sufficient to provoke secondary antibody response.[53,54] Perhaps more sensitive techniques such as immunofluorescence flow cytometry should be used to detect low levels of anti-HLA antibodies in order to exclude 10-20% of patients who are previously alloimmunized[24,25,64] and are unlikely to benefit from the use of leukocyte-depleted blood components. In addition, 40-60% of patients may be immune nonresponders.[64] After eliminating nonresponders and patients with prior alloimmunization, only 20-50% of patients may benefit from the routine use of leukocyte-depleted blood. Additionally, it has been noted that leukemic patients transfused with leukocyte-poor blood experienced a significantly shortened duration of remission than the control group receiving standard components.[65] This finding has prompted concern that a potentially beneficial antileukemic effect may be lost by relying solely on leukocyte-depleted blood components. However, the finding has yet to be confirmed.

Furthermore, the limited amount of data available so far indicate that no more than 5×10^6 leukocytes should be transfused each time in order to ensure the success of preventing primary HLA alloimmunization. Considering the wide range of leukocyte numbers within the same type of blood components and the variability in the extent of leukocyte removal by third-generation filters, stringent quality control using manual counts to detect residual leukocytes becomes essential and adds additional cost to the already expensive third-generation filters.

Currently, an NIH-sponsored multicenter clinical trial to investigate the use of leukocyte-depleted blood components to prevent alloimmunization is being conducted. Before more conclusive scientific data become available from the ongoing study, the routine and indiscriminate use of leukocyte-depleted blood and blood components is premature.

Prevention of Refractoriness to Platelet Transfusion

Refractoriness to platelet transfusion is an extremely complex clinical phenomenon and can be attributed to myriad factors.[66] Although alloimmunization to HLA or other platelet antigens can lead to poor response to platelet transfusion, refractoriness to platelet transfusion also occurs as a result of allosensitization to leukocyte-specific antigens or without any evidence of alloimmunization.[67] Herzig et al[68] reported that the use of leukocyte-depleted platelet concentrates significantly improves platelet transfusion response in those alloimmunized patients who fail to respond to HLA-matched platelet transfusion. Interestingly, all those patients developed leukoagglutinin against donor leukocytes. Their findings suggest that refractoriness to HLA-matched platelet transfusions might result from innocent bystander injury due to the presence of leukoagglutinin against donor leukocytes. Thus, a trial of leukocyte-depleted blood components may be considered when an alloimmunized patient does not respond well to HLA-matched platelet transfusion and there are no identifiable nonimmunological causes.

Prevention of Viral Transmission

Transmission of CMV through blood transfusion to immune-compromised leukemic or aplastic anemia patients can be a major cause of morbidity or mortality, especially in those without history of any prior infection. CMV differs from hepatitis and human immunodeficiency viruses in that it cannot be isolated from plasma.[69] The virus primarily resides in polymorphonuclear leukocytes.[69] Thus, it is reasoned that removal of leukocytes from blood components might prevent CMV infection. Indeed, several studies have shown that the use of leukocyte-poor red cells and platelets is effective to prevent transmission of CMV.[70,71] A further reduction of contaminating leukocytes by using third-generation leukocyte-depletion filters to prevent CMV infection becomes desirable. Recent preliminary studies suggest that the use of leukocyte-depleted blood components can be a suitable alternative to donor screening.[72,73] High-efficiency filters will be valuable in rapidly providing pooled RDP containing unscreened or CMV-positive units for immune-compromised and seronegative patients.

Prevention of Febrile Reactions

Release of endogenous pyrogens from transfused leukocytes activated and/or destroyed by recipient antileukocyte antibodies is the most common mechanism for nonhemolytic febrile transfusion reactions. As reported previously, this reaction occurs in less than 1% of all transfusions and only 15% of patients with previous febrile transfusion reactions experience a second reaction.[74] It is generally accepted that routine use of leukocyte-poor blood components is not warranted unless a patient has repeated febrile reactions. However, patients with leukemia or aplastic anemia require more intensive blood component therapy. Consequently, a much higher percentage of patients will experience recurrent debilitating chills and fevers following blood transfusion. It would be desirable to prevent the febrile transfusion reactions in these patients for their comfort and to avoid confusion with the clinical onset of sepsis.

Since leukocyte-poor blood components, with 90% removal of contaminating white cells, are more than sufficient to prevent most nonhemolytic febrile transfusion reactions,[75] the use of expensive third-generation filters to prepare leukocyte-depleted blood components becomes unnecessary. Moreover, it has been reported that the use of platelet concentrates prefiltered with PL-100® (Pall Corporation, Glen Cove, NY) filters do not significantly reduce the frequency of fever/chill reactions in patients with a history of multiple reactions.[76] This observation supports the view that antileukocyte antibodies are not the only factor responsible for many of the febrile reactions in patients who have received multiple transfusions. Antibodies against platelet-specific antigens or plasma components are also known to be responsible for NHFTR.[63,65-72,77-79] There is no evidence that leukocyte depletion with newly developed third-generation filters is more effective than the use of leukocyte-poor blood components to prevent nonhemolytic febrile transfusion reactions.

Conclusions and Recommendations

All experimental evidence available so far clearly indicates that metabolically active and DR antigen-positive donor leukocytes in blood components are primarily responsible for the initiation of HLA alloimmunization. The results of small-scale clinical studies using leukocyte-depleted blood components to prevent HLA alloimmunization are encouraging. However, rigorous quantitative study for determining a threshold dose of leukocytes necessary to initiate HLA alloimmunization has yet to be completed. The efficacy of leukocyte-depleted blood components for prevention of HLA alloimmunization also needs to be established so that detailed cost/benefit analysis can be performed. In view of the lack of complete scientific data on these issues, indiscriminate use of expensive leukocyte-depleted blood components for all patients with leukemia or aplastic anemia cannot be justified.

In conclusion, the following recommendations are made:

1. The routine use of leukocyte-depleted blood components for prevention of HLA alloimmunization cannot be recommended at this time. The reported data are encouraging but incomplete. The expense for the leukocyte-depletion filter and the necessary quality control is too high to be justified for the uncertain effectiveness. Nevertheless, prevention of HLA alloimmunization can be important for patients who are considered for unrelated allogeneic bone marrow transplantation. If one attempts to prevent HLA alloimmunization by using leukocyte-depleted blood components, patients with evidence of previous alloimmunization should be excluded and careful quality control on the residual number of leukocytes should be performed to ensure that no more than 5×10^6 leukocytes are transfused each time.

2. The use of leukocyte-depleted HLA-matched platelet concentrates may be considered for highly alloimmunized thrombocytopenic patients who do not have other identifiable nonimmunological causes for platelet refractoriness and who respond poorly to HLA-matched platelet transfusion. If there is no improved response, their use should be discontinued.

3. The use of leukocyte-depleted platelet concentrates should be considered for prevention of CMV transmission in severely immune-compromised and seronegative patients, if CMV negative RDPs or SDPs are not readily available.

4. To prevent recurrent nonhemolytic febrile transfusion reactions, removal of leukocytes by using less expensive technology, such as spin-cool-filter for red cells and centrifugation for platelets, is preferred.

Acknowledgment

The authors wish to express their appreciation to Ms. Cathy Smith for her skillful preparation of the manuscript.

References

1. Kicker TS, Bell W, Ness PM, et al. Depletion of white cells from platelet concentrates with a new adsorption filter. Transfusion 1989;29:411-14.
2. Wenz B, Besson N. Quality control and evaluation of leukocyte depleting filters. Transfusion 1989;29:186.
3. Miyamoto M, Sasakawa S, Ishikawa Y, et al. Leukocyte-poor platelet concentrates at the bedside by filtration through Sepacell-PL. Vox Sang 1989;57:164-7.
4. Meryman HT, Hornblower M. The preparation of red cells depleted of leukocytes. Transfusion 1986;26:101-6.
5. Champion AB, Carmen RA. Factors affecting white cell content in platelet concentrates. Transfusion 1985;25:334-8.
6. Slichter SJ. Optimum platelet concentrate preparation and storage. In: Garratty G, ed. Current concepts in transfusion therapy. Arlington, VA: American Association of Blood Banks, 1985:1-26.
7 Skinnider L, Wrohel H, McSheffrey B. The nature of the leukocyte contamination in platelet concentrates. Vox Sang 1985;49:309-14.
8. Sherman ME, Dzik WH. Stability of antigens on leukocytes in banked platelet concentrates. Blood 1988;72:867-72.
9. Koerner K, Kubanek B. Comparison of three different methods used in the preparation of leukocyte-poor platelet concentrates. Vox Sang 1987;53:26-30.
10. Dzik WH. Leukocyte-poor platelet products. In: McCarthy LJ, Baldwin ML, eds. Controversies of leukocyte-poor blood and components. Arlington, VA: American Association of Blood Banks, 1989:49-80.
11. McCullough J, Benson SJ, Yunis EJ, Quie PG. Effect of blood bank storage on leukocyte function. Lancet 1969;2:1333-7.
12. Natali PG, Bigotti A, Nicotra MR, et al. Distribution of human Class I (HLA-A, B, C) histocompatibility antigens in normal and malignant tissues of nonlymphoid origin. Cancer Res 1984;44:4679-46.
13. Bialek JW, Bodmer W, Bodmer J, Payne R. Distribution and quantity of leukocyte antigens in the formed elements of the blood. Transfusion 1966;6:193-204.
14. Kao KJ. Plasma and platelet HLA in normal individuals: Quantitation by competitive enzyme-linked immunoassay. Blood 1987;70:282-6.

15. Van Rood JJ, van Leenwen A, van Santen MCT. Anti-HL-A2 inhibitor in normal serum. Nature 1970;226:366-7.
16. Bach FH, van Rood JJ. The major histocompatibility complex—genetics and biology. N Engl J Med 1976;295:806-13.
17. Zinkernagel RM, Doherty PD. Immunological surveillance against altered self components by sensitized T lymphocytes in lymphocytic choriomeningitis. Nature 1974;251:547-8.
18. Kao KJ, Scornik JC, Riley WJ, McQueen CF. Association between HLA phenotype and HLA concentration in plasma or platelets. Hum Immunol 1988;21:115-24.
19. Schwartz BD. Diversity and regulation of expression of human leukocyte antigen class II molecules. Am J Med 1988;85(Suppl 6A):6-8.
20. Benacerraf B. Significance and biological function of class II MHC molecules. Am J Pathol 1985;120:334-43.
21. Prou O, Kaplan C, Muller JY. Freeze dried platelets for HLA alloimmunization absorption. Tissue Antigen 1980;16:105-7.
22. Howard JE, Perkins HA. The natural history of alloimmunization to platelets. Transfusion 1978;18:496-503.
23. Pamphilon DH, Farrell DH, Donaldson C, et al. Development of lymphocytotoxic and platelet reactive antibodies: A prospective study in patients with acute leukemia. Vox Sang 1989;57:177-81.
24. Eernisse JG, Brand A. Prevention of platelet refractoriness due to HLA antibodies by administration of leukocyte-poor blood components. Exp Hematol 1981;9:77-83.
25. Schiffer CA, Dutcher JP, Aisner J, et al. A randomized trial of leukocyte-depleted platelet transfusion to modify alloimmunization in patients with leukemia. Blood 1988;62:815-20.
26. Fisher M, Chapman JR, Ting A, Morris PJ. Alloimmunization to HLA antigens following transfusion with leukocyte-poor and purified platelet suspensions. Vox Sang 1985;49:331-5.
27. Murphy MF, Metcalfe P, Thomas H, et al. Use of leukocyte-poor blood components and HLA-matched platelet donors to prevent HLA alloimmunization. Br J Haematol 1986;62:529-34.
28. Sniecinski I, O'Donnell MR, Nowicki B, Hill LR. Prevention of refractoriness and HLA alloimmunization using filtered blood products. Blood 1988;71:1402-7.

29. Brand A, Claas FHJ, Voogt PJ, et al. Alloimmunization after leukocyte-depleted multiple random donor platelet transfusions. Vox Sang 1988;54:160-6.
30. Andreu G, Dewailly J, Leberre C, et al. Prevention of HLA immunization with leukocyte-poor packed red cells and platelet concentrates obtained by filtration. Blood 1988; 72:964-9.
31. Claas FHJ, Smeenk RJT, Schmidt R, et al. Alloimmunization against the MHC antigens after platelet transfusion is due to contaminating leukocytes in the platelet suspension. Exp Hematol 1981;9:84-9.
32. Errett LE, Allen N, Deierhoi MH, et al. The effect of platelet transfusions on renal allograft survival and sensitization in dogs. Tissue Antigens 1985;25:28-32.
33. Borleffo JCC, Neuhaus P, van Rood JJ, Blaner H. Platelet transfusion improve kidney allograft in rhesus monkeys without inducing cytotoxic antibodies. Lancet 1982;1: 1117-8.
34. Chapman JR, Ting A, Fisher M, et al. Failure of platelet transfusion to improve human renal allograft survival. Transplantation 1986;41:468-73.
35. Lacy P, Davie J, Finke E. Prolongation of islet allograft survival following in vitro culture (24 C) and a single injection of ALS. Science 1979;204:312-3.
36. Faustman D, Harptfeld V, Lacy P, Davie J. Prolongation of murine islet allograft survival by pretreatment of islets with antibody directed to Ia determinants. Proc Natl Acad Sci USA 1981;78:5156-9.
37. Lau H, Reemtsma K, Hardy MA. Prolongation of rat islet allograft survival by direct ultraviolet irradiation of the graft. Science 1984;223:607-9.
38. Slichter SJ, Deeg HJ, Kennedy MS. Prevention of platelet alloimmunization in dogs with systemic cyclosporine and by UV-irradiation or cyclosporine loading of donor platelets. Blood 1987;69:414-18.
39. Kraemer KH, Levis WR, Cason JC, et al. Inhibition of mixed leukocyte culture reaction by 8-methoxypsoralen and long-wavelength ultraviolet radiation. J Invest Dermatol 1981;77:235-9.
40. Grana NH, Kao KJ. Use of 8-methoxypsoralen (8-MOP) and UV-A pretreated platelet concentrates to prevent alloimmunization against major histocompatibility (MHC) antigens. Blood 1989;74(Suppl 1):215a.
41. Song PS, Tapley KJ. Photochemistry and photobiology of psoralens. Photochem Photobiol 1979;29:1177-97.

42. Cimino GD, Gamper HB, Isaacs ST, Hearst JE. Psoralens as photoactive probes of nucleic acid structure and function. Ann Rev Biochem 1985;54:1151-93.
43. Dinarello CA. Interleukin-1. Ann NY Acad Sci 1988;546: 122-32.
44. Sell S. The immune system. I: Cells and vessels. In: Immunology immunopathology and immunity. New York: Elsevier, 1987:19-36.
45. Kaye J, Hedrick SM. Analysis of specificity for antigen Mls and allogeneic MHC by transfer of T-cell receptor α- and β-chain genes. Nature 1988;336:580-3.
46. van Voorkis WC, Valinsky J, Hoffman E, et al. Relative efficacy of human monocytes and dendritic cells as accessory cells for T cell rejection. J Exp Med 1983;158:174-91.
47. Mizel SB. The interleukins. FASEB J 1989;3:2379-88.
48. Malynn BA, Romeo DT, Worthis HH. Antigen-specific B cells efficiently present low doses of antigen for induction of T cell proliferation. J Immunol 1985;135:980-8.
49. Powers GD, Miller RA. Heterogeneity among T helper cells. J Immunol 1987;139:2567-72.
50. Guy R, Hodes RJ. Antigen-specific, MHC restricted B cell activation by cell free Th2 cell products. J Immunol 1989; 143:1433-40.
51. Lagaaij EL, Hennemann IP, Ruigrok M, et al. Effect of one-HLA-DR antigen matched and completely HLA-DR-mismatched blood transfusions on survival of heart and kidney allografts. N Engl J Med 1989;321:701-5.
52. Pellegrino MA, Indiveri F, Fagiolo V, et al. Immunogenicity of serum HLA antigens in allogeneic combinations. Transplantation 1982;33:530-3.
53. Scornik JC, Ireland JE, Howard RJ, et al. Role of regular and leukocyte-free blood transfusions in the generation of broad sensitization. Transplantation 1984;38:594-8.
54. Everett ET, Kao KJ, Scornik JC. Class I HLA molecules on human erythrocytes: Quantitation and transfusion effects. Transplantation 1987;44:123-9.
55. Pietersz RNI, Dekker WJA, Reesink HW. A new cellulose acetate filter to remove leukocytes from buffy-coat-poor red cell concentrates. Vox Sang 1989;56:37-9.
56. Rydberg L, Ulfrin H, Stigendal L. White cell depletion of platelet concentrates using different filters. Transfusion 1988;28:604-5.
57. Domen RE, Williams L. Use of the Sepacell filter for preparing white cell-depleted red cells. Transfusion 1988;28:506.

58. Pikul FJ, Farrar RP, Boris MB, et al. Effectiveness of two synthetic fiber filters for removing white cells from AS-1 red cells. Transfusion 1989;29:590-5.
59. Saint L, Leitman SF. Use of polyester filter for preparation of leukocyte-depleted platelet concentrates. Blood 1988; 72(Suppl 1):284a.
60. Patten E, Sarala P. Preparation of leukocyte-poor platelet concentrates. Transfusion 1989;29:562-3.
61. Kao KJ, Scornik JC. Accurate quantitation of the low number of white cells in white cell-depleted blood components.Transfusion 1989;29:774-7.
62. Bodensteiner DC. A flow cytometric technique to accurately measure post-filtration white blood cell counts. Transfusion 1989;29:651-3.
63. Murphy MF, Metcalfe P, Ord J, et al. Disappearance of HLA and platelet-specific antibodies in acute leukemia patients alloimmunized by multiple transfusions. Br J Haematol 1987;67:255-60.
64. Dutcher JP, Schiffer CC, Aisner J, Wiernik PH. Long-term follow-up of patients with leukemia receiving platelet transfusions: Identification of a large group of patients who do not become alloimmunized. Blood 1981;58:1007-11.
65. Tucker J, Murphy MF, Gregory WM, et al. Apparent removal of graft-versus-leukemia effect by the use of leukocyte-poor blood component in patients with acute myeloblastic leukemia. Br J Haematol 1989;73:572-81.
66. Bishop JF, McGrath K, Wolf MM, et al. Clinical factors influencing the efficacy of pooled platelet transfusions. Blood 1988;71:383-7.
67. Brubaker DB. Refractoriness to platelet transfusions. J Clin Pathol 1989;91:500-1.
68. Herzig RH, Herzig GP, Bull MI, et al. Correction of poor platelet transfusion responds with leukocyte-poor HLA-matched platelet concentrates. Blood 1975;46:743-50.
69. Adler SP. Transfusion associated cytomegalovirus infections. Rev Infect Dis 1983;5:977-93.
70. Luban NLC, Williams AE, MacDonald MG, et al. Low incidence of acquired cytomegalovirus infection in neonates transfused with washed red blood cells. Am J Dis Child 1987;141:416-9.
71. Murphy MF, Grint PCA, Hadiman AE, et al. Use of leukocyte-poor blood components to prevent primary cytomegalovirus infection in patients with acute leukemia. Br J Haematol 1988;70:253-5.

72. Gilbert GL, Hayes K, Hudson IL, et al. Prevention of transfusion-acquired cytomegalovirus infection in infants by blood filtration to remove leukocytes. Lancet 1989;1:1228-31.
73. Bowden RA, Sayers MH, Cays M, Slichter SJ. The role of blood product filtration in the prevention of transfusion associated cytomegalovirus infection after marrow transplant. Transfusion 1989;29(Suppl):57S.
74. Menitove JE, McElligott MC, Aster RH. Febrile transfusion reaction: What blood component should be given next? Vox Sang 1982;42:318-21.
75. Perkins HA, Payne R, Ferguson J, Wood M. Nonhemolytic febrile transfusion reactions. Quantitative effects of blood components with emphasis on isoantigenic incompatibility of leukocytes. Vox Sang 1966;11:578-600.
76. Chambers LA, Mangano MM, Kruskall MS, et al. Limited efficacy of PL-100 filtration in preventing febrile reactions to platelets. Transfusion 1989;29(Suppl):235.
77. de Rie MA, van der Plas-van Dalen CM, Engelfriet CP, et al. The serology of febrile transfusion reactions. Vox Sang 1958;49:126-34.
78. Barton JC. Non-hemolytic, non-infectious transfusion reactions. Semin Hematol 1981;18:95-121.
79. Dameshek W, Neber J. Transfusion reactions to plasma constituents of whole blood. Blood 1950;5:129-47.

In: Baldwin ML, Kurtz ML and Sirchia G, eds.
Controversies in Transfusion Medicine:
Immune Complications and Cytomegalovirus Transmission
Arlington, VA: American Association
of Blood Banks, 1990

3

Leukocyte-Depleted Blood Components for Patients With Leukemia or Aplastic Anemia—PRO

Marlene M. Fisher, MB, BCh

THERE IS NO LONGER any doubt that blood transfusions have a widespread and prolonged effect on host immunological mechanisms. The consequences can be advantageous or deleterious according to the patient population being studied. The graft protective effect of pretransplant blood transfusion in recipients of renal allografts is well-documented. In more recent years the volume of literature dealing with the deleterious effects has increased alarmingly. These include alloimmunization to histocompatibility antigens, febrile nonhemolytic transfusion reactions, viral transmission, graft-vs-host disease and increased susceptibility to cancer recurrence and postoperative infection. In many instances the harbingers are believed to be "passenger leukocytes," the inevitable and acknowledged constituents of many blood components.

Patients with leukemia and aplastic anemia requiring extensive and protracted transfusion support are particularly vulnerable to transfusion effects, which prejudice the course of the disease. There is growing evidence that leukocyte depletion of blood components would prevent or ameliorate some of the

Marlene M. Fisher, MB, BCh, Deputy Director, Regional Blood Transfusion Centre, John Radcliffe Hospital, Headington, Oxford, England

more damaging consequences of transfusion in these patients. This chapter will summarize the evidence to support this concept, examine the potential for clinical benefit and review the efficiency of current approaches to the provision of leuko-cyte-depleted blood and components.

Leukocyte Mass in Absolute and Relative Terms

"Leukocyte-poor," "leukocyte-depleted" and "leukocyte-free" are ambiguous and misleading terms used to describe blood components that have been modified in some way so that they no longer contain the expected number of leukocytes. The white blood cell content of an unadulterated unit of whole blood is approximately 2.3×10^9 (range $1-5 \times 10^9$)[1] and this is quantitatively split between various blood components according to the production technique used, interval between blood collection and processing, and physiological characteristics of the donor blood. Thus, the leukocyte mass in a single unit of platelets prepared by double spin centrifugation can vary by a factor of 10,[2] and modifications such as buffy coat removal or resuspension in additive media can significantly alter the leukocyte content of red cell suspensions. As the effectiveness of any technique for leukocyte removal depends on the number of leukocytes in the starting material as well as on the method-ology, quality control of leukocyte-depleted components should begin on the production line in the blood bank and continue through to the bedside.

Champion[3] investigated factors that accounted for the wide variation in white cell content of platelet concentrates prepared by double spin centrifugation. The 1 cm of plasma at the red cell interface contained 52% of the leukocyte mass in individ-ual units. By ceasing plasma expression at this level, 22% of the platelets were lost but the component was twice as "pure." Most of the clinical indications for leukocyte-depleted blood components require that a very high proportion of contaminat-ing leukocytes be removed. Currently, "log reduction" is used to quantify the degree of leukocyte depletion relative to the leukocyte mass in the original component and for prevention of alloimunization at least greater than 2 log depletion in a quality blood component is considered to represent an accept-able degree of purity. At this level of depletion, accurate esti-mation of the absolute number of residual leukocytes becomes very difficult and is well below the capacity of automated cell counters, where the limit of accuracy claimed by manufactur-ers is 1000 cells/μL equivalent to 1 log depletion. Modified hemacytometer counts using diluted cell suspensions ensure greater accuracy but are time-consuming and labor-intensive.[4] Flow cytometric techniques appear to provide an excellent means for monitoring the purity of blood components and for testing the efficiency of strategies for leukocyte removal.[5] There is no doubt that as the potential benefits of leukocyte depletion become more widely accepted, the demand for "purity" will increase. Careful clinical evaluation of these components during a new era of improved transfusion support is of crucial importance.

Leukocyte-Poor Blood Components—Potential for Clinical Benefit

Prevention of Alloimmunization

The current approach to chemotherapy in leukemia patients is based on the need to achieve a balance between maximum tumor cell destruction and an acceptable burden of toxicity. It is now clear that in terms of disease-free survival, intensive chemotherapy with several different combinations of drugs used alternatively is a more successful and better tolerated approach than the more prolonged treatment previously favored. Chemotherapy is frequently coupled with allogeneic or autologous bone marrow transplantation and, during periods of severe thrombocytopenia, the availability of histocompatible platelets is of critical importance in the management of these patients.

One of the more serious problems associated with platelet transfusions from multiple random donors is alloimmunization to platelet antigens resulting in poor survival of transfused platelets. Nonavailability of histocompatible donors can preclude administration of effective chemotherapy as there are no proven approaches to the successful management of bleeding in the alloimmunized patient.[6] Any practical means of reducing the incidence of alloimmunization in patients requiring transfusion therapy would be of considerable clinical benefit. Patients are deemed refractory when two consecutive platelet transfusions fail to achieve expected 1-hour and 24-hour posttransfusion platelet increments. This can be secondary to immune destruction or to clinical events that increase platelet consumption such as fever, sepsis, splenomegaly or active bleeding. Alloimmunization can be confirmed serologically by the detection of lymphocytotoxic antibodies directed against histocompatibility antigens of the HLA system and is usually defined as cytotoxicity against >20% of a panel of lymphocytes with broad antigenic representation.[7]

The incidence of alloimmunization documented in the literature varies widely (30-50% to 100%[8]) according to definition of endpoint alloimmunization, heterogeneity of patient population studied and exclusion of risk factors such as previous pregnancy or transfusion. Overall, approximately 40% of new leukemia patients would be expected to become refractory to platelets as a result of alloimmunization within 4-8 weeks of commencement of therapy and irrespective of the number of transfusions administered in that period.[9] Patients with aplastic anemia who have a relatively intact or even enhanced ability to respond to antigen stimuli are reported to have higher rates of alloimmunization (88%) than patients with acute lymphoblastic leukemia (27%).[10]

Measurement of lymphocytotoxic antibody correlates well with responsiveness to random donor platelets. In one study the absence of lymphocytotoxic antibodies was predictive of good transfusion increments in 90% of patients. Poor 24-hour responses in some patients were often explained by antibody at subliminal levels, which could be subsequently demonstrated.[7,11]

Yankee et al[12] first showed that patients refractory to random donor platelets can be successfully treated with platelets from a sibling donor matched for the serologically defined antigens of the HLA system. Due to the polymorphism and complexity of this system, suitable donors are not always found and not all alloimmunized recipients achieve expected increments with HLA-identical platelets. This suggests that non-HLA platelet-reactive antigens can cause destruction of transfused platelets. Pamphilon[13] detected lymphocytotoxic antibody (LCTab) in 20 of 49 patients with acute leukemia, but platelet-reactive antibodies without co-existent LCTab in three patients were not associated with platelet refractoriness. Because of the limitations of the test used, the possibility that some platelet-reactive antibodies were weakly reactive with noncytotoxic LCTab could not be excluded.

In another study, only 7% of patients without demonstrable LCTab did not respond to HLA-compatible platelets.[11] Brand and co-workers[14] found that clinical transfusion failure with HLA perfectly matched platelets occurred in 5 of 335 multitransfused patients as a result of antiplatelet antibody. Only one patient developed platelet-reactive antibody in the absence of LCTab, suggesting that platelet refractoriness to antibodies other than HLA is a rare event and that attempts to modify the immunogenicity of transfused blood components should focus on practical strategies to prevent alloimmunization to HLA antigens.

Histocompatibility antigens—HLA—in humans are controlled by the major histocompatibility complex (MHC) a cluster of genes on the short arm of chromosome 6. They play a central role in T-lymphocyte function in that they associate with foreign antigens to stimulate T cells. There are two types of MHC molecules involved in immune recognition, Class I and Class II. Most nucleated cells express Class I antigens and products of these loci are present on cell surfaces as HLA-A, -B and -C. Class II, expressed as gene products DR, DP and DQ, have a more limited distribution, being present on B cells, macrophages, activated T lymphocytes and some epithelial cells. Antigen-presenting cells (APCs) express both Class I and Class II molecules. An immune response begins with the uptake of antigen by the APC via surface receptors, internal degradation into antigenic peptides and subsequent expression in association with MHC Class II molecules on the cell surface. T cells are activated by this complex via specific T-cell receptors. The precise mechanism by which T lymphocytes recognize *foreign MHC antigens* in tissue grafts such as blood transfusions, is less clear. In this setting, experimental evi-dence suggests that recipient T cells recognize foreign MHC complexed with, possibly, self peptide (ie, it is the donor APCs that present antigen to recipient T-helper cells).[15] If this assumption is correct, one would predict that alloimmunization to MHC antigens would not occur if transfused red cells and platelets were free of viable APCs bearing Class II molecules.

Claas and colleagues[16] were the first to recognize that injection of allogeneic platelets confronts the immune system with a distinctive cell type—platelets being nucleus-free megakaryocytic fragments bearing Class I but not Class II molecules. Using a mouse model to study the effect of variable numbers of contaminating leukocytes on the immunogenicity of platelet suspensions, it was shown that repeated injections of pure platelets failed to initiate a primary immune response to Class I antigen. When 10^3 leukocytes were added, lymphocytotoxic antibodies appeared. Platelets induced a secondary response but it was not clear whether small numbers of residual leukocytes were responsible. Frangoulis[17] confirmed and expanded these observations, reporting that purified platelets depleted of 95% leukocytes did not induce Class I antibody formation or T-cell proliferative responses in murine models, whereas lymphocytes consistently initiated a humoral response even after freezing.

The concept that transfusion of pure platelets would not lead to humoral sensitization and would modify subsequent immune responses was first advocated by Batchelor and Welsh.[18] This view was supported by experimental work in rats,[19] mice,[20] monkeys[21] and mongrel dogs.[22] A report by Borleffs et al[23] that platelet transfusions containing $<10^4$ leukocytes did not sensitize but improved renal allograft survival generated much interest and prompted the first pilot studies in humans. Betuel,[24] using random donor platelets depleted of leukocytes to $<7.6 \times 10^5$ per transfusion, did not sensitize 18 of 19 recipients to HLA antigens and renal allograft survival improved.

Chapman et al[25] used purified platelets to prime 24 previously untransfused patients awaiting their first cadaver renal allograft. The first group of 12 patients received 2×10^{10} platelets (equivalent to 0.5 standard platelet concentrate) containing a mean of 15×10^6 leukocytes per transfusion. A second group of 12 patients received platelets that were further purified by filtration such that leukocyte contamination was below the limits at which it could be measured accurately ($<5 \times 10^6$). Five patients in group 1 developed cytotoxic antibody, whereas in group 2 the pattern of antibody activity did not change. Flow cytometry was used as an adjunct to cytotoxicity assay to detect antibody bound to the surface of platelet donor lymphocytes. Ten patients in group 1 responded to their platelet transfusions as judged by a positive flow cytometry result against T cells from one of their donors; three patients responded to two platelet donors. Only two patients in group 2 showed a weak humoral response.

More recently, Petryani[26] compared the ability of buffy coats and purified platelets to evoke the production of Fc-receptor blocking antibody, which has been associated with improved renal allograft survival. Healthy volunteers were transfused on two occasions with either buffy coat prepared from 400 mL of blood or 10^{10} purified platelets containing $<10^5$ leukocytes. Lymphocytotoxic antibody was detected in three of seven buffy coat recipients and none of five platelet recipients. In contrast to buffy coat transfusions, purified platelets did not induce increased expression of Class II MHC antigen or interleukin-2 receptor on recipient T lymphocytes.[27]

Results of clinical trials where both red cell and platelet suspensions have been rendered leukocyte-depleted are more difficult to interpret than experimental studies involving the use of platelets per se. There are important variables in the data presented by different workers. These include the criteria used to define the refractory state, immune status of patients

Table 3-1. Alloimmunization to Leukocyte-Depleted Blood Components

Author Year (ref)	Patients No.	Patients Type	%+VE HLA Antibodies Control	%+VE HLA Antibodies Leuko-poor	% Refractory Control	% Refractory Leuko-poor	Method of WBC Depletion
Eernisse and Brand 1981(28)	96	leukemia and aplastic anemia	NA 10/14*	NA 12/16*	93% 26/28	24% 16/68	RBCs filtered, >95% depletion (1×10^8)[†]; PCs differential centrifugation 5×10^6/dose
Schiffer 1983(29)	27	leukemia	33% 4/12	27% 4/15	NA	NA -	RBCs frozen (3×10^7)[†] or saline washed (3×10^8)[†]; PCs differential centrifugation 0.12×10^8/pool
Murphy 1986(30)	50	leukemia	48% 15/31	16% 3/19	23% 7/31	5% 1/19	RBCs filtered Imugard 8×10^6/unit; PCs $9\text{-}22 \times 10^7$ apheresis and extra spin
Brand 1988(31)	335	leukemia and aplastic anemia	NA	21% 69[‡]	NA	9% 31/335	RBCs filtered Cellselect 0.5×10^6; PCs differential centrifugation pooled buffy-coat 4-6U, >80%, $<10^7$
Sniecinski 1988(32)	40	leukemia and aplastic anemia	50% 10/20	15% 3/20	50% 10/20	15% 3/20	RBCs filtered Imugard 5×10^7/unit; PCs filtered Imugard 6×10^6/pool
Andreu 1988(33)	69	leukemia and aplastic anemia	31% 11/35	12% 4/34	47% 14/30*	21% 6/28*	RBCs filtered Imugard 0.61×10^8/unit; PCs filtered Imugard 0.47×10^8/pool
Saarinen 1988(34)	35	pediatric oncology	NA	NA	70% 12/17	0% 0/18	RBCs filtered Eurypur 1.0×10^5/unit; PCs filtered Imugard 0.4×10^5/unit

*Number of refractory patients of patients evaluated
[†]Literature value; actual value not documented
[‡]In 18 patients antibodies were transient

studied and number and frequency of transfusions. The results are summarized in Table 3-1. It is difficult to estimate the incidence of refractoriness in nonimmunized patients as not all investigators document this information. Andreu[33] reported four nonimmunized refractory patients in a study group of 28 evaluable recipients of leukocyte-poor transfusions and four in a control group of 30 receiving unmodified blood components. However, the number of patients both immunized and refractory was significantly lower in the leukocyte-poor group, 7% compared with 33%. In another clinical trial the overall incidence of refractoriness in 584 evaluable platelet transfusion events was 11%.[32] In 45% of cases the cause was alloimmunization, the remainder being due either to nonimmune-accelerated consumption or being random events with subsequent transfusions giving adequate increments. Overall, 20-25% of patients became refractory during their first course of chemotherapy but an additional 25% developed signs of refractoriness during consolidation or reinduction therapy up to 18 months later. The time to alloimmunization was significantly less in the control group, as was the number of transfusions received prior to the development of clinical refractoriness.

Attempts by investigators to address the problem of the refractory patient have focused on methods of prevention, circumvention or reversal. The most promising strategy appears to be prevention, either by reducing the number of antigen-presenting cells in blood components, or by modifying the way in which these antigens are presented. Reducing patient exposure to antigen by the use of single donor instead of multiple donor platelets has met with limited success in delaying alloimmunization and inducing a more restricted pattern of antibody formation.[35] However, this approach is costly and would strain the apheresis resources of most transfusion centers. Leukocyte depletion of blood components transfused to patients at risk of alloimmunization provides a simple and convenient alternative. The degree of leukocyte depletion achieved appears to be a critical determinant and overall there is a clear trend toward reduced alloimmunization rates when the level of leukocyte depletion approaches 10^6 (2-3 log removal).

Reduced Incidence of Nonhemolytic Febrile Transfusion Reactions

The commonest event associated with the transfusion of homologous blood components is the nonhemolytic febrile transfusion reaction (NHFTR). The severity of the symptoms varies from mild transient temperature elevation to circulatory collapse and death.[36] In all instances, the NHFTR is a source of apprehension and discomfort to the patient and a cause for concern to the clinician. Although it is recognized that the majority of NHFTRs are immunologically mediated by leukocytes,[37,38] the mechanism that elucidates fever in the recipients is not fully understood. Automated platelet washing, which removes plasma but not leukocytes, eliminated urticarial reactions in strongly alloimmunized patients with leukemia and aplastic anemia but the number of febrile episodes (66% of 301 transfusion reactions) was not reduced.[39]

A significantly large number of patients in the reactor group have HLA alloantibodies, although platelet-specific and granulocyte-specific antibodies have been implicated.[40] The overall incidence has been estimated as 0.5-2.5%, occurring more frequently after granulocyte transfusions (6.49%) than whole blood (0.88%) or platelets (0.4%).[41] However, the NHFTR is the most idiosyncratic and unpredictable of transfusion reactions, as in some patients no cause can be demonstrated, and in others the occurrence and severity vary with each transfusion. de Rie[40] demonstrated HLA antibodies in 66% of reactors compared with 30% in controls. However, antibody screening was performed pretransfusion, whereas Perkins[42] has shown that antibody-negative pretransfusion specimens invariably became positive after transfusion if the patient had experienced a reaction. Thulstrup[43] found evidence of antibodies in all sera of reactors if they were tested against the donor cells responsible for the reaction, but not against cells from donors where no reaction had occurred, suggesting that the reactivity of some antibodies was restricted to antigens of low frequency. The available evidence clearly demonstrates that a high proportion of NHFTRs could be prevented by avoidance of initial sensitization to HLA antigens.

In patients already sensitized, reduction of the absolute number of leukocytes to $<2.5 \times 10^9$ to 0.5×10^9 in red cell transfusion will significantly reduce the incidence of NHFTR.[42] Leukocyte depletion of platelet preparations, however, could mask the signs of developing refractoriness to random donor platelets in strongly alloimmunized recipients. Transfused platelets would be rapidly destroyed by antibodies directed against Class I histocompatibility antigens. As isoimmune destruction of platelets is essentially a silent phenomenon,[44,45] measurement of posttransfusion platelet increments rather than absence of clinical indications of destruction is the most important indicator of the success of platelet therapy in these patients. In an interesting study, Hertzig[46] observed that poor posttransfusion platelet increments to incompatible platelets transfused to leukemia and aplastic anemia patients could be corrected if 96% of contaminating leukocytes were removed by preliminary centrifugation. Posttransfusion increments improved regardless of the HLA match grade between donor and recipient. Although this claim has never been substantiated,[31,47] one could speculate that patients in the early stages of alloimmunization may react less strongly to leukocyte-depleted platelet components due to the lesser expression of HLA antigen on platelets.[48]

Of relevance to this issue is a report by Koskimies[49] that there was progressive disappearance of broadly reactive lymphocytotoxic antibodies in endstage renal patients treated with filtered red cells containing $<2 \times 10^7$ leukocytes. Similar results have been noted in children with chronic anemia where following the use of filtered red cells there was no increase in the potency or spectrum of pre-existing HLA antibodies and, in some instances, antibody activity decreased or disappeared.[50] However, in the absence of clinical data, no firm conclusion can be drawn concerning the efficacy of leukocyte removal in platelet concentrates transfused to strongly alloimmunized patients.

Decreased Risk of Bone Marrow Graft Rejection?

Patients undergoing bone marrow transplantation (BMT) are heavily dependent on transfusion before transplantation because of the nature of the underlying disease, ie, leukemia-lymphoma and aplastic anemia. Graft rejection following BMT is responsible for most of the subsequent morbidity and mortality in patients with aplastic anemia, 24% of rejecting patients becoming long-term survivors compared with 74% with sustained engraftment.[51] The major factors associated with graft failure in these patients include prior blood transfusions, a positive relative response in mixed lymphocyte culture, a low number of cells in the bone marrow inoculum and lack of infusion of viable buffy coats in addition to marrow in transfused patients. The risk associated with prior transfusions is greatest if exposure has been to family members and especially the marrow donor.

Despite extensive blood component therapy during remission induction or consolidation chemotherapy, graft failure is infrequent in patients with leukemia who subsequently receive marrow transplants.[52] The reasons are not clear but may be related to the intensive chemotherapy and radiation regimens used, or to disease-related immunologic unresponsiveness in these patients. In aplastic anemia, graft failure after HLA-identical sibling transplants is assumed to result from immunologic rejection directed at donor minor histocompatibility antigens, although other factors may contribute. The nature of the antigens involved in sensitization and marrow graft rejection is unknown. Experimental studies in canine models suggest that at least two polymorphic minor antigen systems are involved. In one investigation, none of 38 untransfused dogs given a combination of marrow and donor peripheral leukocytes rejected whereas 100% rejection occurred after three transfusions of whole blood from the marrow donor.[53] By comparison, 5 of 14 dogs given transfusions of red blood cells free of leukocytes and platelets rejected the marrow graft and nine had sustained engraftment. The authors speculate that the incidence of rejection after marrow transplantation for aplastic anemia could possibly be reduced if leukocyte-depleted platelets and red cells were used exclusively during the pretransplantation phase.

The observation that the incidence of marrow graft rejection in patients with severe aplastic anemia has decreased in recent years prompted an examination of the changing impact of risk factors. The year of transplant was identified as an independent risk factor for graft rejection[54] as, more recently, pre-graft transfusions represent a less significant risk unless the patient has received large numbers of platelet transfusions (>40). This suggests that changing transfusion practices (ie, fewer whole blood transfusions, lower leukocyte content in blood components and single donor platelets as well as increased shelf life for red cell components) may have contributed to a reduced incidence of marrow rejection. This argument is further substantiated by the fact that the year of transplant is a less significant risk factor in untransfused patients.

A recent multicenter analysis[55] of risk factors for graft failure in 625 patients receiving allogeneic BMT from HLA identical siblings, showed that radiation for pretransplant immunosuppression and use of cyclosporine rather than methotrexate or T-cell depletion of the donor bone marrow, were the major prognostic factors for successful engraftment. However, in 266 patients prepared for transplantation with cyclophosphamide alone, the probability of graft failure was increased in patients who received previous transfusions, with patients who received the highest number of transfusions being at greatest risk.

There are no clinical studies documenting any effect of leukocyte reduction of platelets and red cells in decreasing the incidence of graft rejection in aplastic anemia patients. As these patients are already significantly at risk of other transfusion hazards including latent CMV in circulating lymphocytes, the concept that an optimal transfusion strategy in BMT patients should include the use of leukocyte-depleted blood components deserves further investigation.

Methods for Leukocyte Depletion of Blood Components

Separation of leukocytes from other formed elements in blood can be achieved by exploiting either size/density differences between cells or variations in their surface properties. Low-speed centrifugation sediments cells according to their size, whereas at higher speeds, plasma, platelets, leukocytes and red cells form layers according to their relative densities. Screen/direct interception filters also separate cells by size, acting as mechanical sieves that trap all particles larger than the pores. As removal efficiency is exquisitely dependent on temperature and the extent of spontaneous microaggregate formation in the cell suspension, they are not suitable for separating leukocytes from platelets.[56]

Depth filters, on the other hand, eliminate particles by absorption. They remove discrete populations of cells according to their surface characteristics and the absorptive properties of the filter medium, which can be cotton-wool, polyester or cellulose acetate.

Brittingham and Chaplin[38] were among the first to observe that lowering the leukocyte content of red cells significantly reduced the incidence of nonhemolytic febrile transfusion reactions (NHFTRs). A 1 log reduction of the leukocyte mass in red cell components to $<0.5 \times 10^9$ is indicated for the transfusion of sensitized patients. Techniques that achieve this level of depletion include centrifugation and buffy coat removal, sedimentation, manual and automated cell washing and micro-aggregate filtration.[57] Their effectiveness is limited by density similarities between different populations of cells with consequential high loss of product. The 1 log depletion realized by most of these techniques is less than adequate to avoid primary sensitization to HLA antigens or limit viral transmission.

Centrifugation techniques have also been used to prepare platelet concentrates with a high level of purity.[28] In the right hands, the reported 2 log reduction in leukocyte mass is impressive but quality control of these methods is difficult and platelet loss can be high—20-25%.[58]

Filtration technology has kept pace with the growing interest in purity of blood components. There is a substantial literature documenting the performance characteristics of filters designed for leukocyte depletion of red cell and platelet suspensions in configurations suitable for laboratory or bedside use or both. Manufacturers claim a 2-3 log reduction in leukocyte mass for both red cell and platelet components with concomitant loss of <10% of product. In vitro performance evaluations of depth filters have substantiated these claims in many instances.

Platelet Filters (10^6 residual leukocyte = 2 log reduction)

Kickler[59] filtered (PL100®, Pall Corporation, Glen Cove, NY) 37 platelet pools stored for 2-5 days, each pool consisting of 6, 8 or 10 platelet concentrates. Mean residual white blood cell (WBC) counts of $5.6\text{-}7.5 \times 10^5$ were recorded. After filtration of 10 units, this rose to 9.4×10^5. Platelet loss was 10-15%. Koerner[58] compared filtration (Imugard IG500Y®, Terumo, Tokyo, Japan) with centrifugation techniques for leukocyte removal. Filtration was consistently more efficient; the leukocyte residue in six pooled 2-5-day-old platelet concentrates stored for 2-5 days was $<10^7$. The exact numbers could not be estimated in five experiments as no leukocytes were detected on manual counting. Sepacell PL® (Asahi, Tokyo, Japan) filtration of a 10-unit pool of platelet concentrates reduced the leukocyte mass from 5×10^8 to 2×10^6 with 10% loss of platelets.[60]

Saint[61] compared efficiency of leukocyte depletion in apheresis and pooled multiple donor platelets stored for 1-5 days with Pall PL100 filters. Filtered apheresis products contained a residuum of $<10^6$ WBCs, whereas 50% of pooled multiple donor platelets, which were initially 10 times more heavily contaminated, contained $>10^7$. Rydberg[62] compared Imugard IG500® with Miropoor L® (Travenol Labs, Deerfield, IL). Four to six units of pooled platelets were divided into two portions and filtered. The residual mass of leukocytes was reduced to 10^7 per pool. Platelet loss was 25-30%. Brubaker[63] compared Imugard IG500® with Erypur® (Organon Teknika, Oss, The Netherlands). Ten random donor platelets were pooled and divided, each pool representing a 5-unit dose of platelets.

Automated cell counts for residual WBCs were 3×10^7 for the Erypur® filter and 10^5 for the Imugard filter. The performance of the Erypur® filter was improved by flushing with fresh frozen plasma instead of saline.

Red Cell Filters (10^6 residual leukocyte = 2 log reduction)

Filtration of buffy coat depleted red cells via a Cellselect® (NPBI Emmer Compascwum, The Netherlands) filter reduced the leukocyte mass from 5×10^8 to $<1 \times 10^6$. Red cell loss was approximately 12%.[64] Using an isosmotic ammonium chloride RBC lysis method for counting residual leukocytes in red cells suspended in adenine solution, Pikul[65] estimated the residual WBC mass to be 2.6×10^6 following filtration through a Sepacell® filter. WBC removal was less efficient for second blood units where the residual WBC mass increased to 6.9×10^7. RBC recovery was 95%. Following buffy coat removal and filtration, Sirchia[50] found red cell concentrates to contain $<10^6$ leukocytes in 96% of instances using an Erypur red cell filter and in 65% of instances using an Imugard® filter. In every experiment, the residual leukocyte mass was $<5 \times 10^7$. Both filters were less effective if buffy coat was present.

In performance evaluation of both red cell and platelet filters, the most important considerations are degree of leukocyte removal and concomitant recovery of therapeutic material. Other significant factors include type and immunogenicity of residual cells, clinical effectiveness of final product, capacity of the filter medium for leukocyte removal, cost and practicability. Vakkila[66] used monoclonal antibodies to count and identify subgroups of residual cells in buffy coat depleted red cell concentrates and four-unit pools of platelet concentrates. Comparing the efficiency of three different filters, he reported that the total residual mass of leukocytes per red cell unit was 1.0-8.3×10^5 and for platelet pools 0.4-2.0×10^5. In both instances, less than 3% of the residual cells were Class II MHC antigen-bearing monocytes, which is equivalent to 10^3 cells per product unit. This is well below the estimated threshold for alloimmunization to Class I histocompatibility antigens. The same author showed that the capacity of the Imugard® filter to trap leukocytes decreased significantly when more than four units of platelet concentrates were passed through the filter, possibly because of the low fiber content.

In vitro hemostatic effectiveness of filtered platelets has been investigated by several workers. Measurements of clot retraction, platelet morphology and platelet aggregation to epine-phrine, adenosine diphosphate, collagen or risocetin were un-affected by filtration.[59] In another study, filtered and unfiltered platelets from the same donor were labeled with indium-III and reinfused.[67] There was a slight but statistically significant decrease in survival of the filtered platelets at 6-8 hours but not at 5 days. Cotton-wool filtration of stored platelets ap-peared to have no effect on platelet activation, platelet in vitro function or in vivo percent recovery but caused a slight de-crease in survival hours, which was not considered to be clinically significant.

Of relevance to the timing of leukocyte removal relative to storage of platelet concentrates is the reported influence of WBCs on platelet viability and function. Few laboratory tests have a predictive value for in vivo function of transfused platelets. The most consistently reliable indicator of post-transfusion viability is pH. After storage at pH below 6.0 or above 7.2, transfusion survival is markedly diminished. Beutler and Kuhl[68] reported an inverse relationship between WBC contamination and pH in 20 platelet concentrates stored at room temperature. This finding has been confirmed by other workers[69]: in one investigation variable numbers of leukocytes were added to platelet suspensions in log increments from 10^6-10^9 per platelet concentrate.[70] A significant correlation was found between increasing concentrations of leukocytes and drop in pH, glucose consumption, lactic acid production and release of lactic dehydrogenase. The authors conclude that for optimal storage leukocyte contamination of standard platelet concentrates should not exceed 10^7.

Although the results of in vitro evaluation are encouraging, clinical trials will define the true benefits of the routine use of high performance filters in reducing the incidence of transfu-sion-associated hazards.

Immunomodulation by UV Irradiation

A recent development with exciting possibilities for the future of transfusion therapy is the use of ultraviolet radiation to abrogate the immunizing potential of donor antigen-presenting cells (APCs) in blood components. As long ago as 1971 it was recognized that UV-irradiated white blood cells were unable to proliferate or stimulate allogeneic responder cells in mixed lymphocyte culture.[71] The concept that UV-irradiated platelet concentrates would be incapable of inducing a cellular immune response was supported by experimental evidence in canine models. Only 1 of 12 dogs receiving UV-irradiated platelets was alloimmunized to DLA antigens.[72] The mechanism by which UV light mediates this effect is poorly understood. As described previously, APCs in transfused blood components are responsible for triggering Class II restricted T-helper cell responses. Dendritic cells, unlike other APCs, appear to be constitutive expressors of MHC Class II molecules; APCs also produce molecules that are involved in the activation of lymphocytes. The best characterized is interleukin-1 which acts on T and B cells to potentiate their responses to other lymphokines. When lymphocytes are triggered to proliferate in vitro, they form clusters with dendritic cells before blast formation and proliferation occur. UV-treated dendritic cells have depleted surface expression of Class II molecules and effect decreased T-cell proliferation without reducing the IL-2 expression of these cells. They do not induce cluster formation in vitro.[73] UV light appears to affect Ca++ mobilization in both cell types. Stimulation of T cells with suitable mitogens or monoclonal antibodies against CD3 following UV treatment causes reduced Ca++ release from the endoplasmic reticulum via the second messenger IP3.[74]

UV irradiation, particularly that of intermediate wavelengths (280-320 mn UV-B) inactivates APCS, yet allows normal survival of transfused red cells and platelets.[75] Because of its limited penetration, most plastics are impermeable to UV irradiation and uniform exposure of cells in suspension is difficult to achieve.[76] Concern has also been expressed about the safety of UV irradiation, ie, about UV-induced mutations or activation of latent viruses in transfused cells.[77]

The benefits and drawbacks are yet to be elucidated but immunomodulation of blood components by UV irradiation might prevent graft rejection and anti-host responses in transplantation.

Conclusions and Recommendations

The best method for preventing alloimmunization to histocompatibility antigens has yet to be identified. Immunomodulation of Class II molecules by UV irradiation has great potential but much work needs to be done before pretreatment of blood components becomes routine practice. In the interim, filtration represents the most practical means of reducing the immunogenicity of red cell and platelet components. Leukemia and aplastic anemia patients requiring protracted transfusion support would benefit from such a strategy. High performance filters can reduce the leukocyte mass of blood components to below threshold levels for alloimmunization. Clinical trials show >50% reduction in alloimmunization and refractoriness. The argument that "purified" blood is an extravagance that will benefit only a small proportion of "responders" is difficult to sustain. The cost must be balanced against the considerable financial burden of maintaining panels of HLA-typed apheresis donors to provide histocompatible platelets for alloimmunized patients.[78] Hidden costs such as prolonged hospitalization and donor time must also figure in the equation. Moreover, preliminary observations suggest that the overall requirement for platelets is significantly reduced if filtered components are provided routinely.[34] Finally, there is the ethical dilemma of the bleeding alloimmunized patient for whom no suitable donor can be found.

In patients with leukemia and aplastic anemia treated with bone marrow transplantation, CMV infection is a devastating complication. Once interstitial pneumonitis develops, therapeutic intervention is usually futile. Seronegative blood components are indicated for seronegative recipients but such a policy has been shown to stretch the resources of a blood transfusion center.[79] An optimal transfusion policy of seronegative blood components for all BMT patients and other immunocompromised groups would be logistically impossible. There is ample evidence that CMV is transmitted via the leukocyte fraction in blood components and persuasive evidence that removing this fraction results in reduced or even zero transmission. Filtered blood components from donors of unknown CMV status would provide a practical alternative when seronegative components are not available.

Other benefits of leukocyte-depleted blood components such as reduced risk of transfusion-associated graft-vs-host disease or marrow graft rejection are speculative rather than proven. Leukocyte-poor red blood cells are already indicated for multi-transfused patients experiencing febrile reactions. However, there is no convincing evidence that filtered platelets are of any benefit to broadly alloimmunized patients.

References

1. Merryman HT, Hornblower M. The preparation of red cells depleted of leucocytes. Transfusion 1986;26:101-6.
2. Skinnider L. The nature of the leukocyte contamination in platelet concentrate. Vox Sang 1985;49:309-14.

3. Champion AB, Carmen RA. Factors affecting white cell content in platelet concentrates. Transfusion 1985;25: 334-8.
4. Wenz B. Quality control and evaluation of leukocyte-depleting filters. Transfusion 1989;29:186-7.
5. Bodensteiner DC. A flow cytometric technique to accurately measure post-filtration white blood cell counts. Transfusion 1989;29:651-3.
6. Schiffer CA. Prevention of alloimmunization in platelet transfusion recipients. Platelet immunobiology. Philadelphia: JB Lippincott, 1989:455.
7. Hogge DE, Dutcher JP, Aisner J. Lymphocytotoxic antibody is a predictor of response to random donor platelet transfusion. Am J Hematol 1983;14:363-9.
8. Dutcher JP, Schiffer CA, Aisner J, Wiernik PH. Alloimmunization following platelet transfusion: The absence of a dose response relationship. Blood 1980;57:395.
9. Dutcher JP, Schiffer CA, Aisner J. Long term follow up of patients with leukaemia receiving platelet transfusions: Identification of a large group of patients who do not become alloimmunized. Blood 1981;58:1007-11.
10. Holohan TV, Terasaki PI, Deisseroth AB. Suppression of transfusion-related alloimmunization in intensively treated cancer patients. Blood 1981;58:122-8.
11. Klingemann HG, Self S, Banaji M, et al. Refractoriness to random donor platelet transfusions in patients with aplastic anaemia: A multivariate analysis of data from 264 cases. Br J Haematol 1987;66:115-21.
12. Yankee RA, Grumet RC, Rogentine GN. Platelet transfusion therapy. The selection of platelet compatible donors for refractory patients by lymphocyte HLA typing. N Engl J Med 1969;281:1208-12.
13. Pamphilon DH, Farrell DH, Donaldson C. Development of lymphocytotoxic and platelet reactive antibodies: A prospective study in patients with acute leukaemia. Vox Sang 1989;57:177-81.
14. Brand A, Claas FHJ, Voogt PJ. Alloimmunisation after leukocyte-depleted multiple random donor platelet transfusions. Vox Sang 1988;54:160-6.
15. Marrack P, Kappler J. T cells can distinguish between allogeneic major histocompatibility complex products on different cell types. Nature 1988;332:840-3.
16. Claas FHJ, Smeenk RJT, Schmidt R. Alloimmunization against the MHC antigens after platelet transfusions is due to contaminating leucocytes in the platelet suspension. Exp Hematol 1981;9:84-9.

17. Frangoulis B, Besluau D, Chopin M. Immune response to H-2 class I antigens on platelets. 1. Immunogenicity of platelet class 1 antigens. Tissue Antigens 1988;32:46-54.
18. Batchelor JR, Welsh KI, Burgos H. Immunologic enhancement. Transplant Proc 1977;9:931-6.
19. Welsh KI, Burgos H, Batchelor JR. The immune response to allogeneic rat platelets: Ag-B antigens in matrix form lacking Ia. Eur J Immunol 1977;7:267-72.
20. Weber CJ, Pemis B, Reemtsma K. Donor specific platelet transfusion prolongs mouse islet allograft survival, Transplant Proc 1985;17:1116.
21. Oh JH, McClure HM. Lymphocytotoxic antibodies induced by fresh blood, stored blood and platelets in rhesus monkeys. Transplant Proc 1982;14:410.
22. Errett LE, Allen N, Deierhot MH. The effect of pretransplant platelet transfusions on renal allograft survival and sensitization in dogs. Tissue Antigens 1985;25: 28-32.
23. Borleffs JCC, Neuhaus P, van Rood JJ. Platelet transfusions have a positive effect on kidney allograft survival in rhesus monkeys and induce virtually no cytotoxic antibodies. Transplant Proc 1983;15:985-7.
24. Betuel H, Cantarovitch D, Robert F. Platelet transfusions preparative for kidney transplantation. Transplant Proc 1985;17:2335-7.
25. Chapman JR, Ting A, Fisher M. Failure of platelet transfusion to improve renal allograft survival. Transplantation 1986;41:468-73.
26. Petranyi G, Padanyi A, Horuzsko A. Mixed lymphocyte culture-evidence that pretransplant transfusion with platelets induces FcR and blocking antibody production similar to that induced by leucocyte transfusion. Transfusion 1988:823 4.
27. Takacs K, Szabo T, Kotlan B. In vitro experiments on characteristic changes in functional immune parameters after planned immunization with "buffy coat." Transplant Proc 1986;28:1321-4.
28. Eernisse JG, Brand A. Prevention of platelet refractoriness due to HLA antibodies by administration of leukocyte poor blood components. Exp Hematol 1981;8:77-83.
29. Schiffer CA, Dutcher JP, Aisner J, et al. Randomized trial of leukocyte-depleted platelet transfusion to modify alloimmunization in patients with leukaemia. Blood 1983; 63:815-20.
30. Murphy MF, Metcalfe P, Thomas H, et al. Use of leukocyte-poor blood components and HLA-matched-platelet donors

to prevent HLA alloimmunization. Br J Haematol 1986;62: 529-34.

31. Brand A, Claas FHJ, Voogt PJ, et al. Alloimmunisation after leukocyte-depleted multiple random donor platelet transfusions. Vox Sang 1988;54:160-6.

32. Sniecinski I, O'Donnell MR, Nowicki B. Prevention of refractoriness and HLA-alloimmunisation using filtered blood products. Blood 1988;71:1402-7.

33. Andreu G, Dewailly J, Leberre C, et al. Prevention of HLA immunisation with leucocyte poor packed red cells and platelet concentrates obtained by filtration. Blood 1988; 72:964-9.

34. Saarinen UM, Kekomaki R, Siimes MA, et al. Effective go prophylaxis against platelet refractoriness in multi-transfused patients: Use of leukocyte-free blood components (abstract). Proceedings of the April 1988 Meeting of the American Society of Clinical Oncology. Philadelphia: WB Saunders, 1988:281.

35. Gmur J, von Felten A, Osterwalder B. Delayed alloimmunisation using random single donor platelet transfusions: A prospective study in thrombocytopaenic patients with acute leukaemia. Blood 1983;62:473-9.

36. Menitove JE, McElligott MC, Aster RH. Febrile transfusion reactions: What blood should be given next? Vox Sang 1982;42:318-21.

37. Payne R. The association of febrile transfusion reactions with leucoagglutinins. Vox Sang 1957;2:233.

38. Brittingham TE, Chaplin H. Febrile transfusion reactions caused by sensitivity to donor leukocyctes and platelets. JAMA 1957;165:819.

39. Buck SA, Kickler TS, McGuire HG. The utility of platelet washing using an automated procedure for severe platelet allergic reaction. Transfusion 1987;27:391-3.

40. de Rie MA, van der Plas-van Dalen CM, Engelfreit CP, et al. The serology of febrile transfusion reactions. Vox Sang 1985;49:126-34.

41. Decary F, Ferner P, Giavedoni L, et al. An investigation of non-haemolytic transfusion reactions. Vox Sang 1984;46: 277-85.

42. Perkins HA, Payne R, Ferguson J, Wood M. Non-haemolytic febrile transfusion reactions: Quantitative effects of blood components with emphasis on isoantigenic incompati-bility of leucocytes. Vox Sang 1966;11:578-600.

43. Thulstrup H. The influence of leucocyte and thrombocyte incompatibility on non-haemolytic transfusion reactions 1. A retrospective study. Vox Sang 1971;21:233-50.

44. Van de Wiel ThWM, Van de Wiel-Dorfmeyer H, van Loghem JJ. Studies on platelet antibodies in man. Vox Sang 1961; 6:641.
45. Dausset J, Colin M, Colombani J. Immune platelet isoantibodies. Vox Sang 1960;5:4.
46. Hertzig RH, Hertzig GP, Bull MI, et al. Correction of poor platelet transfusion responses with leukocyte poor HLA matched platelet concentrates. Blood 1975;46:743-50.
47. Slichter SJ. Controversies in platelet transfusion therapy. Ann Rev Med 1980;31:529.
48. Szatkowski NS, Aster RH. HLA antigens on platelets IV. Influence of private HLA-B locus specificities on the expression of Bw4 and Bw6 on human platelets. Tissue Antigens 1980;15:361-8.
49. Koskimies S, Julin M, Ahonen J. Follow up of cytotoxic antibodies in sensitized patients waiting for a kidney transplant: Impact of leukocyte-free blood transfusions. Transplant Proc 1986;28:20-2.
50. Sirchia G, Parravicini A, Rubella P, et al. Effectiveness of red blood cells filtered through cotton-wool to prevent antileukocyte antibody production in multitransfused patients. Vox Sang 1982;42:190-7.
51. Storb R, Prentice RL, Thomas ED, et al. Factors associated with graft rejection after HLA identical marrow transplantation for aplastic anaemia. Br J Haematol 1983;55:573-85.
52. Ho WG, Champlin RE, Winston DJ, et al. Bone marrow transplantation in patients with leukaemia previously transfused with blood products from family members. Br J Haematol 1987;67:67-70.
53. Storb R, Weiden PL, Deeg HJ, et al. Rejection of marrow from DLA-identical canine littermates given transfusions before grafting: Antigens involved are expressed on leukocytes and skin epithelial cells but not on platelets and red blood cells. Blood 1979;54:477-84.
54. Deeg HJ, Self S, Storb R, et al. Decreased incidence of marrow graft rejection in patients with severe aplastic anaemia: Changing impact of risk factors. Blood 1986;68:1363-8.
55. Champlin RE, Horowitz MM, Van Bekkum DW, et al. Graft failure following bone marrow transplantation for severe aplastic anaemia: Risk factors and treatment results. Blood 1989;73:606-13.
56. Snyder EL, de Palma L, Napychank P. Use of polyester filters for the preparation of leukocyte poor platelet concentrates. Vox Sang 1988;54:21-3.

57. Merryman HT, Hornblower M. The preparation of red cells depleted of leukocytes. Transfusion 1986;26:101-6.
58. Koerner K, Kubanek B. Comparison of three different methods used in the preparation of leukocyte poor platelet concentrates. Vox Sang 1987;53:26-30.
59. Kickler TS, Bell W, Ness PM, et al. Depletion of white cells from platelet concentrates with a new adsorption filter. Transfusion 1989;29:411-4.
60. Miyamoto M, Sasakawa S, Ishikawa Y, et al. Leukocyte poor platelet concentrates at the bedside by filtration through Sepacell-PL. Vox Sang 1989;57:164-7.
61. Saint L, Leitman SF, Davey RJ. Use of a polyester filter for preparation of leukocyte depleted platelet concentrates (abstract). Blood 1988;72(5)Suppl 1:284a.
62. Rydberg L, Ulfvin A. White cell depletion of platelet concentrates using different filters (letter). Transfusion 1988; 28:605.
63. Brubaker DB, Romine CM. The in vitro evaluation of two filters (Erypur and Imugard Ig 500) for white cell poor platelet concentrates. Transfusion 1988;28:383-5.
64. Pietersz RMI, Reesink HW, de Korte D, et al. Storage of leukocyte poor red cell concentrates: Filtration in a closed system using a sterile connection device. Vox Sang 1989; 57:29-36.
65. Pikul F, Farrar R, Marlo D, et al. In-line polyester fibre filtration produces "leukocyte free" red blood cells for transfusions (abstract). Transfusion 1987;27:531.
66. Vakkila J, Myllylä G. Mount and type of leukocytes in "leukocyte free" red cell and platelets concentrates. Vox Sang 1987;53:76-82.
67. Holme S, Ross D, Heaton WA. In vitro and in vivo evaluation of platelet concentrates after cottonwool filtration. Vox Sang 1989;57:112-15.
68. Beutler E, Kuhl W. Platelet glycolysis in platelet storage IV. The effect of supplementary glucose and adenine. Transfusion 1980;20:97-100.
69. Gottschall JL, Johnston VJ, Rzad L, et al. Importance of white blood cells in platelet storage. Vox Sang 1984;47: 101-7.
70. Pietersz RNI. Leukocyte poor platelet concentrates. A new method for routine preparation. Amsterdam: Free University Press, 1988.
71. Lindahl-Kiessling K, Safwenberg J. Inability of UV irradiated lymphocytes to stimulate allogeneic cells in mixed lymphocyte culture. Int Arch Allergy Appl Immunol 1971; 41:670-8.

72. Slichter SJ, Deeg HJ, Kennedy MS. Prevention of platelet alloimmunisation in dogs with systemic cyclosporine and by UV irradiation or cyclosporine loading of donor platelets. Blood 1987;69:414-18.

73. Aprile J, Deeg HJ. Ultraviolet irradiation of canine dendritic cells prevents motogen-induced cluster formation and lymphocyte proliferation. Transplantation 1986;42: 653-60.

74. Berridge MJ. Inositol triphosphate and diacylglycerol: Two interacting second messengers. Ann Rev Biochem 1987; 56:159-93.

75. Kahn RA, Duffy BF, Rodey GG. Ultraviolet irradiation of platelet concentrate abrogates lymphocyte activation without affecting platelet function in vitro. Transfusion 1985; 25:547-50.

76. Deeg HJ, Aprile J, Graham TC, et al. Ultraviolet irradiation of blood prevents transfusion-induced sensitization and marrow graft rejection in dogs. Blood 1986;67:537-9.

77. Deeg HJ. Transfusions with a tan. Prevention of allosensitization by ultraviolet irradiation. Transfusion 1989;29: 450-5.

78. Freedman J, Gafni A, Garvey B, Blanchette V. A cost-effective evaluation of platelet crossmatching and HLA matching in alloimmunised thrombocytopenic patients. Transfusion 1989;29:201-7.

79. Bowden RA, Sayers M, Gleaves M, et al. Cytomegalovirus-seronegative blood components for the prevention of primary cytomegalovirus infection after marrow transplantation. Transfusion 1987;27:478-81.

In: Kurtz SR, Baldwin ML and Sirchia G, eds
*Controversies in Transfusion Medicine:
Immune Complications and Cytomegalovirus Transmission*
Arlington, VA: American Association
of Blood Banks, 1990

4

Irradiation of Blood Components To Prevent Graft-vs-Host Disease

Kenneth C. Anderson, MD and Howard J. Weinstein, MD

GRAFT-VS-HOST DISEASE (GVHD) is commonly observed after allogeneic bone marrow transplantation (BMT) but rarely recognized posttransfusion (PT) or following solid organ transplantation.[1-3] Posttransfusion GVHD usually occurs in the immunosuppressed recipient (eg, premature newborns, infants with congenital immunodeficiency syndromes and patients with leukemia or lymphoma), but recent reports also involve immunocompetent recipients.[4-10] Although the pathophysiology of GVHD remains to be fully elucidated, the clinical manifestations are well appreciated in the appropriate clinical setting (ie, after allogeneic BMT). This syndrome is characterized by fever and skin rash, which usually begins as an erythematous maculopapular eruption centrally, spreads to the extremities and may progress to generalized erythroderma and bullous formation in severe cases. Additional manifestations may include anorexia, nausea, vomiting and watery or bloody diarrhea with or without elevated liver enzymes and hyperbilirubinemia. Since there are no pathognomonic features of GVHD, this syndrome is sometimes difficult to distinguish from viral infections or drug eruptions. Immunosuppressive therapies such as prednisone, antithymocyte globulin and cyclosporine have been used to treat post-BMT GVHD but have not been effective for GVHD-PT.

Kenneth C. Anderson, MD, Medical Director, Blood Component Laboratory, Dana-Farber Cancer Institute and Assistant Professor of Medicine, Harvard Medical School; Howard J. Weinstein, MD, Associate Professor of Pediatrics, Harvard Medical School, Boston, Massachusetts

GVHD-PT is usually severe, akin to the situation in HLA-mismatched BMT and frequently results in pancytopenia secondary to marrow aplasia. The majority of cases of GVHD-PT are fatal.

Clinical and laboratory data indicate that the transfusion of immunocompetent T lymphocytes into an immunodeficient allogeneic recipient is a requisite for the development of GVHD. Although risk factors for post-BMT GVHD have been defined,[11] the degree and type of recipient immunodeficiency that predisposes to GVHD-PT are largely unknown. Cases continue to develop in immunocompromised as well as immunocompetent hosts. Moreover, the lack of reported GVHD after transfusion of unirradiated blood components to patients who are known to be immunodeficient (ie, those with acquired immune deficiency syndrome and those who have undergone organ transplantation) further suggests that this syndrome may be underrecognized, or that risk factors predisposing to GVHD remain undefined.

Potentially useful measures to prevent GVHD-PT include gamma irradiation or depletion of T lymphocytes from blood components before transfusion. Prevention of the harmful effects of transfusion by irradiation of blood has been in routine use by marrow transplant teams for more than two decades[12] and, to date, no cases of GVHD-PT have been reported in recipients of irradiated blood components. In contrast, leukocyte depletion techniques to prevent GVHD are unproven. This review will critically examine the reported experience of GVHD-PT in order to: 1) define those individuals at risk for this syndrome and 2) assess current modalities for its prevention and treatment.

Historical Perspective

Graft-vs-host disease was originally described following transfusion in immunodeficient children in 1965.[13] During the next 15 years, 38 cases of GVHD-PT were described in these clinical settings: severe combined immunodeficiency (SCID) and Wiskott-Aldrich (WA) syndromes; newborns with erythroblastosis fetalis (EF); and patients with hematologic malignancies including Hodgkin's disease (HD) and non-Hodgkin's lymphoma (NHL), acute lymphoblastic and myelocytic leukemia (ALL and AML) and chronic lymphocytic leukemia (CLL).[4] Exchange transfusion and intrauterine transfusion as well as transfusion of whole blood, packed red blood cells (PRBCs), buffy coats (BCs), granulocytes (WBCs) harvested from both normal donors and from patients with chronic myelocytic leukemia, and platelets (Plts) have all been implicated in cases of GVHD-PT. Although its true incidence remained unknown, in 1982 GVHD-PT was estimated to occur in 0.1-1.0% of patients with hematologic malignancies or lymphoproliferative diseases.[4] At that time, patients with Hodgkin's disease who had a prolonged history of treatment, all patients with malignancies who were treated with several remission induction programs, all patients with immunodeficiency syndromes and neonates with ery-throblastosis fetalis were felt to be at risk for GVHD-PT and, therefore. candidates to receive transfusion of irradiated blood components.

Since the Von Fliedner review,[4] the number of reported cases of this syndrome has increased and the spectrum of patients at risk has broadened, but its true incidence remains unde-fined. In 1984, Weiden recommended that irradiated intra-uterine or exchange transfusions should be given for hemolytic disease of the newborn, and that irradiated blood component transfusions should also be given to patients with acute leu-kemia, neuroblastoma, Hodgkin's disease and non-Hodgkin's lymphoma (particularly those being treated with chemotherapy or radiotherapy); to patients with severe congenital or acquired immune deficiencies; and to those receiving marrow trans-plants.[14] It was also at this time that GVHD-PT was described following blood transfusion in a patient who had surgery for an aortic aneurysm and was not recognized to be immunocom-promised.[15] Nonetheless, the provision of irradiated blood com-ponents to all patients with congenital or acquired immu-nodeficiency remained controversial. Lind, for example, in 1985 suggested that this stance might be premature, citing the fact that several important features were as yet undefined: the true incidence of GVHD-PT; the groups at risk for the compli-cation; its spectrum of clinical presentations; and the efficacy of methods utilized to prevent it.[16] Moreover, he emphasized the clinical and budgetary consequences of sanctioning a po-tentially unnecessary clinical practice without additional care-ful reporting of its incidence and characteristics, examination of its effects upon different groups of patients and initiation of studies to determine whether its prevention would affect pa-tient care.

In 1987, Kessinger and colleagues described posttransfu-sion GVHD in a patient with Hodgkin's disease and reviewed 27 other reported cases of GVHD-PT in patients with both hematologic malignancies (acute leukemia and lymphoma) and solid tumors (neuroblastoma, rhabdomyosarcoma and glio-blastoma).[6] All transfusion recipients had received cytotoxic chemotherapy, and 13 had received prior radiation therapy. In spite of attempts at therapy of GVHD-PT, the majority (82%) of patients died. These authors concluded that the incidence of GVHD-PT is probably low, but that the lack of response to treatment should prompt consideration of efforts to prevent it.

Until recently, GVHD-PT had been reported in patients with solid tumors only rarely, primarily in the setting of intensive therapy for neuroblastoma.[17,18] However, GVHD-PT was reported in four of 34 patients with solid tumors (three lung cancers and one germ cell cancer) who were treated with high doses of chemotherapy and autologous marrow infusions and subsequently received transfusions of nonirradiated blood cells.[19] Moreover, additional cases of GVHD-PT have also been documented in patients with Hodgkin's disease who were treated with chemotherapy alone.[20,21] It appears that combined radiation therapy and chemotherapy are not necessary as predisposing factors. Finally, a recent report documents GVHD-PT in a patient with cervical carcinoma, further expanding the spectrum of patients with solid tumors who appear to be at risk.[22]

Two cases of GVHD-PT have recently been documented in premature infants who received unirradiated blood components.[23,24] One received RBC transfusions in the setting of hyaline-membrane disease and ventricular hemorrhages, and the other received RBCs and WBCs in the setting of suspected sepsis and respiratory distress syndrome. It is important to emphasize that neither of these infants had congenital immunodeficiency syndromes or erythroblastosis fetalis, which are recognized risk factors for the development of GVHD-PT.

GVHD-PT also continues to be reported in individuals without obvious immunodeficiencies. A recently reported survey[15] of 340 hospitals in Japan documented 96 cases of postoperative erythroderma in 63 of the 257 patients who underwent cardiac surgery between 1981 and 1986, with a mortality rate of 90%. Although HLA typing was reported for only 3 of these cases, this syndrome appears to be identical to GVHD-PT.[15,25,26] A single case of GVHD-PT after cardiac surgery has been reported in the United States.[8] Thaler and colleagues have recently reported two cases of fatal GVHD-PT in immunocompetent adult patients after cardiac surgery.[9] Both received transfusions of fresh, nonirradiated whole blood from their children. In each case, one of the blood donors was HLA-homozygous for one of the recipient's haplotypes. Fatal GVHD has also recently been reported in a woman after cholecystectomy who received a transfusion of RBCs from a donor homozygous for an HLA haplotype shared by the recipient.[10] In this setting, the donor lymphocytes are not recognized by the recipient (no host-vs-graft) and react against HLA antigens encoded by the recipient's other haplotype. Finally, another report documents fatal GVHD-PT occurring in a 22-year-old woman who received two units of blood transfused after delivery.[27] This patient had only mild pre-eclampsia, was not immunocompromised and therefore not felt to be at risk for GVHD-PT.

Who Is at Risk?

The true incidence of posttransfusion GVHD presently remains unknown. Moreover, the spectrum of patients at risk for the development of GVHD-PT has not yet been clearly defined. To date, graft-vs-host disease has been reported after transfusion of unirradiated blood components to at least 87 patients: in patients with severe combined immunodeficiency, thymic hypoplasia and Wiskott-Aldrich syndrome; premature newborns and those with erythroblastosis fetalis[13,23,24,28-43]; patients with hematologic malignancies including Hodgkin's and non Hodgkin's lymphomas, acute myelocytic and lymphoblastic leukemias, chronic lymphocytic leukemia and aplastic anemias[4,6,20,21,44-68]; patients with solid tumors including neuroblastoma, glioblastoma, rhabdomyosarcoma, cervical carcinoma, small cell lung cancer and germ cell tumor[17-19,22,69]; patients after cardiac surgery and cholecystectomy[8-10,15,22]; and in an apparently healthy 22-year-old woman[27] (Tables 4-1 through 4-4). This syndrome has developed following exchange and intrauterine transfusions and after transfusion of whole blood, plasma, red blood cells, platelets and leukocytes harvested from normal donors and from donors with chronic myelocytic leukemia.

The most common manifestations of GVHD-PT include rash, abnormal liver function tests and severe pancytopenia. GVHD-PT results in an overall 84% mortality after a median of 21 (8-1050) days. Although the mortality may be less in patients with leukemias (50%, Table 4-3) than in other subgroups of patients (96-100%) (Tables 4-1, 4-2 and 4-4), there is to date no evidence that any therapy for GVHD-PT influences the outcome. The degree of pancytopenia is generally much more profound in this setting than after GVHD associated with allogeneic BMT. In the setting of GVHD-PT, hematopoiesis is of recipient origin and, therefore, susceptible to attack by donor T cells. In contrast, hematopoiesis is of donor origin and affected to a lesser extent by GVHD after allogeneic BMT.

Table 4-1. Posttransfusion Graft-vs-Host Disease in Patients With Immunodeficiency Syndromes and in Newborns

Patient	Age*	Sex†	Disease‡	Product Transfused§	Outcome‖	Day After Transfusion	Reference
1	3.5 m	M	SCID	ET(WB)	D	17	13
2	11 m	M	SCID	WB	D	28	29
3	3 m	M	SCID	WB	D	17	37
4	5 m	M	SCID	plasma	D	14	37
5	3 m	M	SCID	WB	D	20	30
6	4 m	M	SCID	WB/RBC	D	16	40
7	5 m	M	SCID	WB	D	12	33
8	11 y	M	SCID	plasma	S	—	35
9	term	M	SCID	WB	D	28	43
10	18 m	M	SCID	RBC	D	15	34
11	16 m	M	thymic hypoplasia	plasma	D	29	39
12	8 m	F	thymic hypoplasia	BC	D	14	13
13	32 wg	M	WA	plasma	D	30	31
14	33 wg	M	EF	IU/ET	D	91	32
15	36 wg	M	EF	IU(RBC)/ET(WB)	D	12	36
16	36 wg	F	EF	IU(RBC)/ET(WB)	D	19	36
17	32 wg	M	EF	IU(RBC)/ET(WB)	D	21	38
18	term	M	EF	ET(WB)	D	20	38
19	term	F	EF	ET(WB)	D	80	42
20	33 wg	M	P	ET/RBC/Plt	D	36	41
21	28 wg	M	P	ET/(WB)	D	120	28
22	25 wg	F	P	RBC/	D	42	23
23	28 wg	F	P	RBC/WBC	D	46	24

*Months(m), days(d), years(y) of age or weeks gestation(wg)
†Male(M) or female(F)
‡Severe combined immunodeficiency syndrome (SCID), Wiskott-Aldrich syndrome (WA), erythroblastosis fetalis (EF), premature infants (P)
§Whole blood (WB), red blood cells (RBC), buffy coat (BC), exchange transfusion (ET), intrauterine transfusion (IU), normal granulocytes (WBC)
‖Died(D) or survived(S)

Table 4-2. Posttransfusion Graft-vs-Host Disease in Patients With Lymphoma

Patient	Age (yrs)	Sex*	Disease†	Product Transfused‡	Outcome§	Day After Transfusion	Reference
1	30	F	HD	CML WBC	S	—	44
2	28	F	HD	CML WBC	D	31	44
3	30	F	HD	WB	D	15	45
4	21	F	HD	RBC	D	21	45
5	24	M	HD	WB/Plt	D	12	46
6	31	M	HD	Plt	D	12	4
7	18	F	HD	RBC	D	25	47
8	5	M	HD	WBC	D	29	48
9	21	F	HD	Plt	D	27	49
10	37	F	HD	RBC/Plt	D	23	49
11	61	F	HD	RBC	D	47	6
12	14	M	HD	Plt	D	32	20
13	20	F	HD	RBC	D	38	20
14	—	—	HD	RBC/Plt	D	8	21
15	—	—	HD	RBC/Plt	D	8	21
16	14	M	NHL	CML WBC	D	8	44
17	20	M	NHL	RBC/Plt	D	2	46
18	34	M	NHL	WBC	D	24	50
19	6	M	NHL	BC	D	13	51
20	18	F	NHL	WBC	D	22	52
21	30	F	NHL	WBC	D	63	53
22	50	F	NHL	RBC	D	43	54
23	20	M	NHL	WB/Plt	D	22	55

*Male(M) or female(F)
†Hodgkin's disease (HD) or non-Hodgkin's lymphoma (NHL)
‡Whole blood (WB), red blood cells (RBC), platelets (plt), chronic myelocytic leukemia granulocytes (CML WBC), normal granulocytes (WBC) or buffy coat (BC)
§Died(D) or survived(S)

Table 4-3. Posttransfusion Graft-vs-Host Disease in Patients With Leukemia and Aplastic Anemia

Patient	Age (yrs)	Sex*	Disease†	Products Transfused‡	Outcome§	Day After Transfusion	Reference
1	50	M	AML	WBC/Plt	D	19	56
2	15	F	AML	CML WBC	S	—	57
3	—	—	AML	CML WBC	S	—	57
4	6	M	AML	RBC/WBC/Plt	S	—	58
5	60	M	AML	RBC/WBC/Plt	D	18	59
6	45	M	AML	RBC/WBC/Plt	D	45	59
7	19	M	AML	RBC/Plt	D	30	60
8	38	M	AML	RBC/WBC/Plt	S	—	60
9	49	M	AML	WB/WBC	D	—	61
10	49	M	AML	RBC/WBC	D	—	61
11	15	M	AML	WB/RBC/Plt	D	—	61
12	5	M	ALL	WB	D	—	62
13	5	M	ALL	CML WBC	S	—	44
14	20	F	ALL	CML WBC	S	—	44
15	15	M	ALL	CML WBC	S	—	44
16	7	F	ALL	WBC	D	18	63
17	5	F	ALL	WBC	S	—	64
18	5	M	ALL	CML WBC	S	—	65
19	61	F	ALL	CML WBC	S	—	66
20	5	F	ALL	WB	D	1050	67
21	10	M	ALL	WBC	S	—	67
22	54	F	CLL	CML WBC	S	—	66
23	12	F	AA	CML WBC	D	—	57
24	34	F	AA	WB	D	—	68

*Male(M) or female(F)
†Acute myelocytic leukemia (AML), acute lymphoblastic leukemia (ALL), chronic lymphocytic leukemia (CLL) or aplastic anemia (AA)
‡Granulocytes (WBC), platelets (Plt), chronic myelocytic leukemia granulocytes (CML WBC), red blood cells (RBC), whole blood (WB)
§Died (D) or survived (S)

Table 4-4. Posttransfusion Graft-vs-Host Disease in Patients With Solid Tumors, Patients After Cardiac Surgery and Individuals Without Known Risk Factors

Patient	Age (yrs)	Sex*	Disease†	Product Transfused‡	Outcome§	Day After Transfusion	Reference
1	59	F	GB	BC	D	12	48
2	2	M	NB	RBC	D	21	17
3	2	F	NB	RBC	D	13	18
4	9	F	RM	RBC/Plt	D	24	69
5	56	F	cervical ca	RBC	D	17	22
6	53	M	SCLC	RBC/Plt	D	—	19
7	55	M	SCLC	RBC/Plt	D	—	19
8	53	M	SCLC	Plts	D	26	19
9	25	F	GC	WBC	D	9	19
10	66	F	CS	WB	D	16	22
11	68	M	CS	WB	D	—	15
12	44	M	CS	WB	D	—	15
13	63	M	CS	RBC	D	26	8
14	69	M	CS	WB	D	22	9
15	51	M	CS	WB	D	34	9
16	52	F	C	RBC	D	28	10
17	22	F	P	RBC	D	28	27

*Male (M) or female (F)

†Neuroblastoma (NB), glioblastoma (GB), rhabdomyosarcoma (RM), small cell lung cancer (SCLC), germ cell tumor (GC), cardiac surgery (CS), normal pregnancy (P), cholecystectomy (C)

‡Red blood cells (RBC), granulocytes (WBC), platelets (Plt), buffy coat (BC), whole blood (WB)

§Died (D) or survived (S)

Factors Predisposing to GVHD-PT

Transfusions during gestation and to newborns, premature infants and infants with congenital immunodeficiency syndromes may result in GVHD-PT due to the underlying immunocompromised status of the recipients. Patients with hematologic malignancies and solid tumors may be immunosuppressed secondary to either chemotherapy and/or radiation therapy but may also have intrinsic immune dysfunction (eg, Hodgkin's disease).[70] As therapeutic approaches for malignancy have become more intensive (ie, high dose chemotherapy followed by autologous bone marrow transplantation), there will be an increasing number and spectrum of individuals at risk for GVHD-PT.[71-73] In such cases, it will be important to document that the GVHD is related to a transfused product, since mild GVHD has been documented in patients who underwent either autologous or syngeneic marrow grafting and received only irradiated blood components.[74]

It is interesting that there have been no reported cases of GVHD-PT in patients with acquired immunodeficiency syndrome (AIDS). Perhaps some of the signs and symptoms (rashes, pancytopenia, liver function abnormalities) presently attributed to infections, drug reactions and other coexistent medical conditions in patients with AIDS may well be related to GVHD-PT, since it is not yet uniform policy to provide irradiated blood components to these individuals. Finally, GVHD-PT has only rarely been reported in recipients of organ transplants other than bone marrow, or in patients on immunosuppressive medications for autoimmune or other diseases. A more heightened awareness on the part not only of hematologists and oncologists but also physicians and health-care providers generally, coupled with prompt reporting of cases of GVHD-PT, is essential to define its true incidence and the spectrum of patients who are at risk.

It has been suggested that transfusion from donors homozygous for an extended haplotype to a recipient sharing this extended haplotype may predispose to GVHD-PT[75] analogous to Thaler's case report from Israel.[9] Although there is extreme polymorphism of alleles in the HLA system, a small number of haplotypic combinations of MHC markers between HLA-B and HLA-DR comprise nearly 30% of common haplotypes and are called extended haplotypes.[76] It has been shown that reactivity in mixed lymphocyte culture between unrelated individuals matched for common extended haplotypes is as low as that between MHC-identical siblings.[77] The probability that blood from donors homozygous for any extended haplotype might be transfused to recipients heterozygous for the same extended haplotype is quite high in Caucasians (about 1 in 500 transfused). If this is true, why don't we see more GVHD-PT? Other factors such as the number and viability of transfused lymphocytes and host defenses must play a role. Nonetheless, these data may have implications for transfusion policy more generally. "Directed donations" are often utilized currently, although without proven benefit, to improve the safety of blood transfusions. Often these donors are family members who could share HLA antigens (a single haplotype or more) with the recipients, thus predisposing to the development of GVHD-PT. As is well-known, the provision of HLA-matched platelets, those from donors sharing at least two antigens at the HLA-B and B loci, has been demonstrated to result in satisfactory platelet increments in alloimmunized patients refractory to standard platelet transfusion therapy.[78] In this setting, it is also possible that the provision of platelets from donors sharing HLA antigens may predispose to GVHD-PT.

Strategies for Prevention of Graft-vs-Host Disease Posttransfusion

Since attempts at treatment of GVHD-PT have not been successful, the primary emphasis has been on prevention. Two methods are currently available that could potentially be utilized to avoid GVHD-PT: gamma irradiation and depletion of leukocytes from blood components prior to transfusion. Prevention of the harmful effects of transfusion by irradiation of blood was first described in mice in 1959[79] and in man 2 years later.[80,81] It has been in routine use by marrow transplant teams for more than 2 decades.[12] It has been shown that as little as 500 rad of gamma irradiation can abrogate the response of lymphocytes to allogeneic cells in a mixed lymphocyte culture, and 1500 rad can reduce response to mitogen-induced stimulation by 90%.[82,83]

Moreover, Button and colleagues[84] have examined the function of blood components after irradiation doses of 500 to 20,000 rad and demonstrated that doses as high as 5000 rad decreased mitogen stimulation by 98.5%, but did not compromise function of cells other than lymphocytes. Specifically, irradiated red blood cells had the same survival as nonirradiated controls; granulocytes had normal in vitro bacterial killing capacity, chemotactic mobility and superoxide production; and transfused irradiated platelets produced the expected increases in platelet counts and controlled hemostasis in thrombocytopenic patients. In this study, however, doses of 5000 rad decreased the yield of platelets posttransfusion by one third. Based upon this and other studies of the effects of gamma irradiation on in vitro cell function and posttransfusion recovery, it has been recommended that the lowest dose capable of inhibiting lymphocyte proliferation be utilized to irradiate blood components prior to transfusion—1500-2500 rad.[5,82-89] The paucity of cases of GVHD-PT after transfusion of irradiated blood components confirms the efficacy of this approach.

Recently, a patient with chronic myelogenous leukemia who received a T-cell depleted histocompatible marrow allograft developed both graft rejection and graft-vs-host disease.[90] Cytogenetic, restriction fragment length polymorphism and DNA-based HLA typing using polymerase chain reaction confirmed that cells in peripheral blood and marrow were neither those from the donor nor recipient. Despite the fact that all blood components were irradiated with 2000 rad, these cells were felt to represent a population of proliferating transfused cells that were alloreactive against both donor and host. Moreover, studies using limiting dilution suggest that the frequency of irradiated lymphocytes able to respond to mitogen is reduced by 5-6 logs by irradiation at 1500 to 2000 rad, compared to irradiated controls.[90] However, a small percentage of lymphocytes may survive irradiation at these doses, suggesting that existing blood component irradiation guidelines may require reassessment.

Several studies address the potential adverse consequences of irradiation, including release of potassium into irradiated stored blood. Ramirez and colleagues irradiated red cell concentrates at 3000 rad immediately after collection, stored them under standard conditions and noted a threefold elevation in potassium levels relative to controls.[91] Rivet and colleagues confirmed that potassium levels increase with length of storage in both irradiated and nonirradiated red cell concentrates, that the length of storage prior to irradiation does not significantly affect the potassium level and that manual washing and reconstitution with fresh frozen plasma were effective in reducing the potassium levels of all red cell concentrates.[92] The extent of potassium release has led to the recommendation that blood required for intrauterine, neonatal or pediatric transfusion not be stored after irradiation,[91] or that irradiated red cell concentrates used for neonatal transfusions be washed manually to reduce potassium levels.[92] Others have suggested that the total infusion load of potassium is so low that it is not clinically significant.[93] For the adult transfusion recipient, in fact, the amount of potassium release is clinically insignificant; however, the difference of almost two orders of magnitude in the plasma volume of adults and newborns makes a clinically insignificant amount of potassium in an adult a substantial load in a neonate.[91,92,94,95] Thus, irradiated components should be washed prior to intrauterine, neonatal or pediatric transfusion.

The second potential method to prevent GVHD-PT would be to deplete lymphocytes from blood components prior to transfusion. It has been demonstrated in murine systems, as well as in man, that T lymphocytes mediate GVHD and that the incidence and severity of GVHD postallogeneic BMT can be reduced if T cells are eliminated from the donor marrow prior to grafting by a variety of techniques.[96,97] Most currently utilized ex vivo methods for T-cell depletion remove >90% of T cells from donor marrow, with approximately 10^7 residual marrow T lymphocytes (10^5-10^6/kg recipient body weight).[98-101] Although these techniques abrogate GVHD in HLA-matched patients, almost every study reports at least some patients who develop GVHD, with more severe GVHD in HLA- mismatched patients. While it may not be either possible or practical to treat blood components in a similar fashion, techniques are presently available for the depletion of leukocytes from red cells: elimination of buffy coat after centrifugation; direct or inverted dilution-centrifugation; washing; cotton or cellulose acetate filtration; or freezing.[102] Leukocytes can be removed from platelets by centrifugation and cotton or acetate filtration.[103-106] To date these efforts have evolved for the avoidance of leukocyte-related transfusion reactions or alloimmu-nization, and are under investigation for viral depletion. However, since the number and precise T cells required to mediate GVHD-PT remain undefined, it is unknown whether depletion of leukocytes using these currently available techniques would decrease the risk of GVHD-PT. It is known that frozen blood contains less than 2% residual leukocytes with intact proliferative ability,[102] confirming that some immunocompetent T cells are present and suggesting that this currently employed leukocyte depletion technique may not be effective prophylaxis against GVHD-PT. Although the incidence of GVHD could be significantly decreased with the development of more effective leukocyte depletion techniques, at present these techniques are expensive, time-consuming and of unproven value. Simple in vitro irradiation accomplishes the desired goal inexpensively, rapidly and with proven efficacy.

Recently, a canine model has been used to demonstrate that ultraviolet (UV) rather than gamma irradiation of transfused leukocytes can abrogate GVHD in recipient animals.[107] Specifically, 10 dogs were given 9.2 cGy of total body irradiation and autologous bone marrow infusion followed by 10 daily trans-fusions of leukocytes for a median total of 18.8 (11.5-36.2)/kg. All four dogs that received unirradiated leukocytes, two of three dogs given leukocytes irradiated with 20 mJ/cm² ultraviolet light (200-300 min) and none of 3 dogs transfused with leu-kocytes irradiated to 1000 mJ/cm² developed GVHD. Prelimi-nary studies in man have utilized UV irradiation of blood components to minimize alloimmunization.[108] Future studies will determine whether treatment with UV light can, in fact, prevent either alloimmunization or GVHD-PT in transfusion recipients without adverse effects on in vitro function or in vivo recovery of UV-treated red cells or platelets.

Conclusion and Recommendations

Graft-vs-host disease after transfusion continues to be re-ported in individuals at known risk for this complication and also in those recipients who are not thought to be immunodefi-cient. The former reflects a lack of awareness of this complica-tion by hematologists, oncologists and others caring for known immunodeficient hosts, and the latter highlights our lack of knowledge of the extent of immunodeficiency necessary to predispose to GVHD-PT. More generalized recognition of this syndrome, prompt reporting of all such cases and studies of the recipient's immune status may allow more precise cat-egorization of individuals at risk. A 1986 National Institutes of Health consensus conference defined patients who have un-dergone bone marrow transplantation or those with other forms of immunodeficiency as candidates for irradiated platelet concentrates to prevent GVHD.[109] At present, within our spe-cialized setting of caring for patients with malignancies, we have recently recommended that all such patients receive irradiated blood components to avoid this complication. Some other cen-ters caring for similar patients are also tending toward this view, but it cannot at present be more widely justified. If sporadic reports of GVHD-PT continue in the fu-ture, irradiation of blood components prior to transfusion may be more generally useful in transfusion medicine practice. This may be especially true in the clinical settings of known ac-quired immunodeficiency states, such as with AIDS or after organ trans-plantation.

The recent cases of GVHD-PT reported after cardiac surgery in both Israel and Japan[9,15] occurred after transfusion of fresh whole blood, utilized due to the purported improved hemostatic effect of fresh whole blood versus platelet concentrates; how-ever, there is no evidence that fresh blood is in fact more useful in this regard than stored blood.[110,111] Moreover, there is no evidence that avoidance of the transfusion of fresh blood components can prevent GVHD. Indeed, some components, ie, platelets, must be used "fresh" or after only 5 days of storage. At present, therefore, there is no reason to alter storage time between donation and transfusion of blood components due to concern for GVHD-PT.

The GVHD-PT syndrome appears to be more likely if donor and recipient share a common haplotype. Indeed, the specialized setting recently reported from Israel[9] involved an HLA homozygous donor who shared a recipient haplotype. The homogeneity of the Israeli population and, [....therefore, the likelihood of....] having an extended haplotype-homozygous donor may explain the more frequent reports of GVHD-PT in these immunocompetent recipients. Directed donations from immediate family members may also increase the likelihood of GVHD-PT because such donors would share HLA antigens with recipients. Thaler and colleagues in Israel have discontinued the use of fresh blood from patients' family members and believe that the chance that randomly selected, unrelated donors will be HLA-homozygous and share haplotypes is so low that GVHD-PT is highly unlikely to develop. Alternatively, irradiation of blood components from such "directed" donations may be utilized to avoid this complication. Indeed, since homozygosity for HLA types is more likely to occur among first degree family members (ie, parents, children and siblings), patient directed donations may therefore carry a risk of initiating GVHD-PT. The American Association of Blood Banks has, therefore, recently recommended that cellular blood components from such donors be irradiated with at least 1500 rad prior to transfusion.[112]

In the United States, the major method to prevent GVHD-PT is gamma irradiation of the product prior to transfusion, as it is unclear whether any manipulation of blood components prior to transfusion could deplete the effector cells of GVHD sufficiently to abrogate this syndrome. The technology is presently available for irradiation of blood components, and such irradiation appears to have no adverse effects on red cell, granulocyte or platelet function in vitro or on in vivo recovery and function of these cells after transfusion.

Acknowledgment

The author would like to thank Ms. Bernadette Miner for her secretarial assistance.

References

1. Storb R, Deeg HJ, Fisher L, et al. Cyclosporine vs methotrexate for graft-versus-host-disease prevention in patients given marrow grafts for leukemia: Long term follow-up of three controlled trials. Blood 1988;71:293-8.
2. Transfusion and graft-versus-host disease (editorial). Lancet 1989;1:529-30.
3. Burdick JF, Vogelsang GB, Smith WJ, et al. Severe graft-versus-host disease in a liver transplant recipient. N Engl J Med 1988;318:689-91.
4. Von Fliedner V, Higby DJ, Kim U. Graft versus host reaction following blood transfusion. Am J Med 1982; 72:951-6.
5. Leitman SF, Holland PV. Irradiation of blood products: Indications and guidelines. Transfusion 1985;25:293-300.
6. Kessinger A, Armitage JO, Klassen LW, et al. Graft versus host disease following transfusion of normal blood products to patients with malignancies. J Surg Oncol 1987; 36:206-9.
7. Holland PV. Prevention of transfusion-associated graft-vs-host disease. Arch Pathol Lab Med 1989;113:285-91.
8. Arsura EL, Bertelle A, Minkowitz S, et al. Transfusion-associated-graft-versus-host disease in a presumed immunocompetent patient. Arch Intern Med 1988;148: 1941-4.
9. Thaler M, Shamiss A, Orgad S, et al. The role of blood from HLA-homozygous donors in fatal transfusion-associated graft-versus-host disease after open heart surgery. N Engl J Med 1989;321:25-8.
10. Otsuka S, Kunieda K, Hirose M, et al. Fatal erythroderma (suspected graft-versus-host disease) after cholecystectomy. Transfusion 1989;29:544-8.
11. Bross DS, Tutschka J, Farmer ER, et al. Predictive factors for acute graft-versus-host-disease in patients transplanted with HLA-identical bone marrow. Blood 1984;63:1265-70.
12. Thomas ED, Storb R, Clift RA, et al. Bone marrow transplantation. N Engl J Med 1975;192:832-43, 895-902.
13. Hathaway WE, Githens JH, Blackburn WR, et al. Aplastic anemia, histiocytosis and erythrodermia in immunologically deficient children. N Engl J Med 1965;273:953-8.
14. Weiden P. Graft-vs-host disease following transfusion. Arch Intern Med 1984;144:1557-8.

15. Sakakibara T, Juji T. Post-transfusion graft-versus-host disease after open heart surgery. Lancet 1986;2:1099.
16. Lind SE. Has the case for irradiating blood products been made? Am J Med 1985;78:543-4.
17. Woods WG, Lubin BH. Fatal graft-versus-host disease in a child with neuroblastoma. Pediatrics 1981;67:217-21.
18. Kennedy JS, Ricketts RR. Fatal graft versus host disease in a child with neuroblastoma following a blood transfusion. J Ped Surg 1986;21:1108-9.
19. Postmus PE, Mulder NH, Elema JD. Graft versus host disease after transfusions of non-irradiated blood cells in patients having received autologous bone marrow. Eur J Cancer Clin Oncol 1988;24:889-94.
20. DeCoste SD, Boudreaux C, Dover JS. Transfusion-associated graft-versus-host disease in patients with malignancies: report of two cases and review of the literature. Arch Dermatol 1990 (in press).
21. Ekert H, Waters KD, Smith PJ, et al. Treatment with MOPP or Ch1VPP chemotherapy only for all stages of childhood Hodgkin's disease. J Clin Oncol 1988;6:1845-50.
22. Matsushita M, Shibata Y, Fuse K, et al. Sex chromatin analysis of lymphocytes invading host organs in transfusion-associated graft-versus-host disease. Virchows Arch [B] Cell Pathol 1988;55:237-9.
23. Sanders M, Graeber J, Zehnbauer B, et al. Post-transplant graft-versus-host disease in a premature infant without known risk factors (abstract). Blood 1988; 72 (Suppl 1):384a.
24. Berger RS, Dixon SL. Fulminant transfusion-associated graft-versus-host disease in a premature infant. J Am Acad Derm 1989;20:945-50.
25. Ito K, Yoshida H, Yanagibashi K. Change of HLA phe-notype in postoperative erythroderma. Lancet 1988;1: 413-4.
26. Juji T, Takahashi K, Shibata Y, et al. Post transfusion graft-versus-host disease in immunocompetent patients after cardiac surgery. N Engl J Med 1989;321:56.
27. Sheehan T, McLaren KM, Brettle R, Parker AC. Transfusion-induced graft versus host disease in pregnancy. Clin Lab Haematol 1987;9:205-7.
28. Hathaway WE, Brangle RW, Nelson TL, Roekel IE. Aplastic anemia and alymphocytosis in an infant with hypo-gammaglobulinemia: Graft versus host reaction? J Pediatr 1966;68:713-22.

29. Hathaway WE, Fulginiti VA, Pierce CW, et al. Graft versus host reaction following a single blood transfusion. JAMA 1967;201:1015-20.
30. Jacobs JC, Blanc WA, de Capoa A, et al. Complement deficiency and chromosomal breaks in a case of Swiss-type agammaglobulinemia. Lancet 1968;1:499-503.
31. Douglas SD, Fudenberg HH. Graft versus host reaction in Wiskott-Aldrich syndrome: Antemortem diagnosis of human GVH in an immunologic deficiency disease. Vox Sang 1969;16:172-8.
32. Naiman JL, Punnett HH, Lischner HW, et al. Possible graft-versus-host reaction after intrauterine transfusion for erythroblastosis fetalis. N Engl J Med 1969;281:697-701.
33. Gatti RA, Platt N, Pomerance HH, et al. Hereditary lymphogenic agammaglobulinemia associated with a distinctive form of short-limbed dwarfism and ectodermal dysplasia. J Pediatr 1969;75:675-84.
34. Robertson WRC, Berry CL, Macaulay JC, Soothill JF. Partial immunodeficiency and graft versus host disease. Arch Dis Child 1971;46:571-4.
35. Rubinstein A, Radl J, Cottier H, et al. Unusual combined immunodeficiency syndrome exhibiting kappa-IgD paraproteinemia, residual gutimmunity and graft-versus-host reaction after plasma infusion. Acta Paediatr Scand 1973;62:365-72.
36. Parkman R, Mosier D, Umansky I, et al. Graft versus host disease after intrauterine and exchange transfusions for hemolytic disease of the newborn. N Engl J Med 1974;290:359-63.
37. Park BH, Good RA, Gate J, Burke B. Fatal graft-versus-host reaction following transfusion of allogeneic blood and plasma in infants with combined immunodeficiency disease. Transplant Proc 1974;6:385-7.
38. Bohm N, Kleine N, Enzel U. Graft-versus-host disease in two newborns after repeated blood transfusions because of Rhesus incompatibility. Beitr Path Vol 1977;160:381-400.
39. McCarty JR, Raimer SS, Jarratt M. Toxic epidermal necrolysis from graft-vs-host disease. Occurrence in a patient with thymic hypoplasia. Am J Dis Child 1978;132:282-4.
40. Niethammer D, Goldmann SF, Flad HD, et al. Graft-versus-host reaction after blood transfusion in a patient with cellular immunodeficiency: The role of histocompatibility testing. Eur J Pediatr 1979;132:43-8.

41. Seemayer TA, Bolande RP. Thymic involution mimicking thymic dysplasia. A consequence of transfusion-induced graft versus host disease in a premature infant. Arch Pathol Lab Med 1980;104:141-4.
42. Lauer BA, Githens JH, Hayward AR, et al. Probable graft-vs-host reaction in an infant after exchange transfusion and marrow transplantation. Pediatrics 1982;70: 43-7.
43. Brouard J, Morin M, Borel B, et al. Di Georges syndrome complicated by graft versus host reaction. Arch Fr Pediatr 1985;42:853-5.
44. Mathe G, Schwarzenberg L, DeVries MJ, et al. Les divers aspects du.syndrome secondaire compliquant les transfusions allogeniques de moelle osseuse ou de leukocytes chez des sujets atteints d'hemopathies malignes. Eur J Cancer 1965;1:75-113.
45. Schaerer R, Schaerer L, Sotto JJ, et al. La reaction du greffon contre l'hote (GVHR) comme complication detale des transfusions de sang au cours de la maladie de Hodgkin: a propos de deux observations (abstract). Proc Premier Congres Francais d'Hematologie, Vittel, 1975.
46. Groff P, Torhorst J, Speck B, et al. Graft versus host disease, a little known complication of blood transfusions. Schweiz Med Wochenschr 1976;106:634-9.
47. Dinsmore RE, Strauss DJ, Pollack MS, et al. Fatal graft-versus-host disease following blood transfusion in Hodgkin's disease documented by HLA typing. Blood 1980; 55:831-4.
48. Schmidmeier W, Feil W, Gebhart W, et al. Fatal graft-versus-host reaction following granulocyte transfusions. Blut 1982;45:115-19.
49. Burns LO, Westberg MW, Burns CP, et al. Acute graft-versus-host disease resulting from normal donor blood transfusion. Acta Haematol 1984;71:270-6.
50. De Dobbeleer GD, Ledoux-Corbusier MH, Achten GA. Graft versus host reaction. An ultrastructural study. Arch Dermatol 1975; 11:1597-602.
51. Betzhold J, Hong R. Fatal graft-versus-host disease after a small leukocyte transfusion in a patient with lymphoma and varicella. Pediatrics 1978;62:63-6.
52. Weiden PL, Zuckerman N, Hansen JA, et al. Fatal graft-versus-host disease in a patient with lymphoblastic leukemia following normal granulocyte transfusions. Blood 1981;57:328-32.

53. Tolbert B, Kaufman CE, Burgdorf WHC, Brubaker DB. Graft-versus-host disease from leukocyte transfusions. J Am Acad Dermatol 1983;9:416-19.
54. Gossi U, Bucher U, Brun del Re G, et al. Acute graft-versus-host disease following a single transfusion of erythrocytes. Schweiz Med Wochenschr 1985;115:34-40.
55. Saab GA, Kurban AK, Mutasim DF. Graft-versus-host disease in lymphoblastic lymphoma following blood transfusions. Middle East J Anesthesiol 1983;7:221-5.
56. Ford JM, Lucey JJ, Cullen MH, et al. Fatal graft versus host disease following transfusion of granulocytes from normal donors. Lancet 1976;2:1167-9.
57. Lowenthal RM, Grossman L, Goldman JM, et al. Granulocyte transfusions in treatment of infections in patients with acute leukemia and aplastic anemia. Lancet 1975;1:353-8.
58. Cohen D, Weinstein H, Mihm M, Yankee R. Nonfatal graft-versus-host disease occurring after transfusion with leukocytes and platelets obtained from normal donors. Blood 1979;53:1053-7.
59. Lowenthal RM, Menon C, Challis DR. Graft-versus-host disease in consecutive patients with acute myeloid leukemia treated with blood cells from normal donors. Aust NZ J Med 1981;11:179-83.
60. Schmitz N, Kayser W, Gassmann W, et al. Two cases of graft versus host disease following transfusion of nonirradiated blood products. Blut 1982;44:83-8.
61. Nikoskelainen J, Soderstrom K-O, Rajamaki A, et al. Graft-versus-host reaction in 3 adult leukaemia patients after transfusion of blood cell products. Scand J Haematol 1983;31:403-9.
62. Berkel AI, Tinaztepe K. Graft-versus-host reaction manifested as toxic epidermal necrolysis in a patient with acute leukemia. Turk J Pediatr 1981;23:37-41.
63. Rosen RC, Huestis DW, Corrigan JJ. Acute leukemia and granulocyte transfusion: Fatal graft-versus-host reaction following transfusion of cells obtained from normal donors. J Pediatr 1978;93:268-70.
64. Salfner B, Borberg H, Kruger G, et al. Graft-versus-host reaktion nach granulozyten transfusion von einen Normalspender. Blut 1978;36:27-34.
65. Schwarzenberg L, Mathe G, Amiel JL, et al. Study of factors determining the usefulness and complications of leukocyte transfusions. Am J Med 1967;43:206-13.
66. Mathe G, Amiel JL, Schwarzenberg L. Bone marrow transplantation and leukocyte transfusions. In: Kugel-

mass IN, ed. Bone marrow transplantation. Springfield, Illinois: CC Thomas, 1971:119-25.

67. Siimes MA, Koskimies S. Chronic graft-versus-host disease after blood transfusions confirmed by incompatible HLA antigens in bone marrow (letter). Lancet 1982;1:42.

68. Wechsler A, Magnin PH, Casas JG, et al. Post-transfusion graft vs host reaction in aplastic anemia. Med Cutan Ibero Lat Am 1984;12:203-7.

69. Labotka RJ, Radvany R. Graft-versus-host disease in rhabdomyosarcoma following transfusion with nonirradiated blood products. Med Pediatr Oncol 1985;13:101-4.

70. Twomey JJ, Rice L. Impact of Hodgkin's disease upon the immune system. Semin Oncol 1980;7:114-25.

71. Cheson BD, Lacerna L, Leyland-Jones B, et al. Autologous bone marrow transplantation. Current status and future directions. Ann Intern Med 1989;110:51-65.

72. Armitage RJ, Goldstone AH, Richards JDM, Cawley JC. Lymphocyte function after autologous bone marrow transplantation (BMT): A comparison with patients treated with allogeneic BMT and with chemotherapy only. Br J Haematol 1986;63:637-47.

73. Rappeport J, Parkman R, Anderson K, Sullivan K. Immunological reconstitution post bone marrow transplantation and late infectious complications. In: McArthur JR, ed. Hematology 1988. Philadelphia: Grune and Stratton, 1988:81-4.

74. Hood AF, Vogelsang GB, Block LP, et al. Acute graft versus host disease development following autologous and syngeneic bone marrow transplantation. Arch Dermatol 1987;123:745-50.

75. Kruskall MS, Alper CA, Awdeh Z, Yunis EJ. HLA-homozygous donors and transfusion-associated graft-versus-host disease (letter). N Engl J Med 1990;322: 1005-6.

76. Awdeh ZL, Raum D, Yunis EJ, Alper CA. Extended HLA/complement allele haplotypes: Evidence for T/t like complex in man. Proc Natl Acad Sci USA 1983;80:259-63.

77. Awdeh ZL, Alper CA, Eynon E, et al. Unrelated individuals matched for MHC extended haplotypes and HLA-identical siblings show comparable responses in mixed lymphocyte culture. Lancet 1985;2:853-6.

78. Yankee RA, Grumet FC, Rogentine GN. Platelet transfusion therapy. The selection of compatible platelet donors for refractory patients by lymphocyte HLA typing. N Engl J Med 1969;281:1208-12.

79. Cole LJ, Garver RM. Abrogation by injected mouse blood of the protective effect of foreign bone marrow in lethally x-irradiated mice. Nature 1959;184:1815-6.

80. Goodman JW, Congdon CC. The killing effect of blood-bone marrow mixtures given to irradiated mice. Radiat Res 1960;12:439-40.

81. Thomas ED, Herman EC Jr, Greenough III WB, et al. Irradiation and marrow infusion in leukemia. Arch Intern Med 1961;107:829-45.

82. Sprent J, Anderson RE, Miller JFAP. Radiosensitivity of T and B lymphocytes. II. Effect of radiation on response of T cells to alloantigens. Eur J Immunol 1974;4:204-10.

83. Valerius NH, Johansen KS, Nielson OS, et al. Effect of in vitro x-irradiation on lymphocyte and granulocyte function. Scand J Hematol 1981;27:9-18.

84. Button LN, DeWolf WC, Newburger PE, et al. The effects of irradiation on blood components. Transfusion 1981; 21:419-26.

85. Holley TR, Van Epps DE, Harvey RI, et al. Effect of high doses of radiation on human neutrophil chemotaxis, phagocytosis, and morphology. Am J Pathol 1974;75:61-8.

86. Patrone F, Dallegri F, Brema F, Sacchetti C. Effects of irradiation and storage on granulocytes harvested by continuous-flow centrifugation. Exp Hematol 1979;7: 131-6.

87. Buescher ES, Gallin JI. Leukocyte transfusions in chronic granulomatous disease. N Engl J Med 1982;307:800-3.

88. Read EJ, Kadis C, Carter CS, et al. Viability of platelets following storage in the irradiated state. A pair-controlled study. Transfusion 1988;28:446-50.

89. Rock G, Adams GA, Labow RS. The effects of irradiation on platelet function. Transfusion 1988;28:451-5.

90. Drobyski W, Thibodeau S, Truitt RL, et al. Third party mediated graft rejection and graft-versus-host disease after T cell depleted bone marrow transplantation, as demonstrated by hypervariable DNA probes and HLA-DR polymorphism. Blood 1989;74:2285-94.

91. Ramirez AM, Woodfield DG, Scott R, McLachlan J. High potassium levels in stored irradiated blood (letter). Transfusion 1987;27:444-5.

92. Rivet C, Baxter A, Rock G. Potassium levels in irradiated blood (letter). Transfusion 1989;29:185.

93. Ferguson DJ. Potassium levels in irradiated blood (letter). Transfusion 1989;29:749.

94. Rock G, Shear JM. Potassium levels in irradiated blood (letter). Transfusion 1989;29:749.

95. Bernard DR, Chapman RG, Simmons MA, et al. Blood for use in exchange transfusions in the newborn. Transfusion 1980;20:401-8.

96. Sprent J, Von Boehmer H, Nabholz M. Association of immunity and tolerance to host H-2 determinants in irradiated F1 hybrid mice reconstituted with bone marrow cells from one parental strain. J Exp Med 1975; 142:321-31.

97. Korngold R, Sprent J. T cell subsets and graft-versus-host disease. Transplantation 1987;44:335-9.

98. Filipovich AH, Vallèra DA, Youle RJ, et al. Graft-versus host-disease prevention in allogeneic bone marrow transplantation from histocompatible siblings: A pilot study using immunotoxins for T cell depletion of donor bone marrow. Transplantation 1987;44:62-9.

99. Anderson KC, Nadler LM, Takvorian T, et al. Their use in bone marrow transplantation. In: Brown E, ed. Progress in hematology. Orlando: Grune and Stratton, 1987:137-81.

100. Reisner Y, Kapoor N, Kirkpatrick D, et al. Transplantation for acute leukaemia with HLA-A and B nonidentical parental marrow cells fractionated with soybean agglutinin and sheep red blood cells. Lancet 1981;2:327-31.

101. de Witte T, Hoogengout J, de Pauw B, et al. Depletion of donor lymphocytes by counterflow centrifugation successfully prevents acute graft-versus-host-disease in matched allogeneic marrow transplantation. Blood 1988; 5:1302-8.

102. Crowley JP, Skrabut EM, Valeri CR. Immunocompetent lymphocytes in previously frozen washed red cells. Vox Sang 1974;26:513-17.

103. Schiffer CA, Dutcher JP, Aisner J, et al. A randomized trial of leukocyte depleted platelet transfusion to modify alloimmunization in patients with leukemia. Blood 1983; 62:815-20.

104. Eernisse JG, Brand A. Prevention of platelet refractoriness due to HLA antibodies by administration of leucocyte-poor blood components. Exp Hematol 1981;9:77-83.

105. Murphy MF, Metcalfe P, Thomas H, et al. Use of leukocyte-poor blood components and HLA matched platelet donors to prevent HLA alloimmunization. Br J Haematol 1986;62:529-34.

106. Sniecinski I, O'Donnell MR, Nowicki B, Hill LR. Prevention of refractoriness and HLA-alloimmunization using filtered blood products. Blood 1988;71:1402-7.
107. Deeg HJ, Graham TC, Gerhard Miller L, et al. Prevention of transfusion-induced graft-versus-host disease in dogs by ultraviolet irradiation. Blood 1989;74:2592-5.
108. Brand A, Claas FHJ, van Rood JJ. UV-irradiated platelets: Ready to use? Transfusion 1989;29:377-8.
109. NIH consensus conference. Platelet transfusion therapy. JAMA 1987;257:1777-80.
110. Mohr R, Martinowitz Y, Lavee J, et al. The hemostatic effect of transfusing fresh whole blood versus platelet concentrates after cardiac operations. J Thorac Cardiovasc Surg 1988;96:530-4.
111. Wasser MN, Houblers JG, D'Amaro J, et al. The effect of fresh versus stored blood on post-operative bleeding after coronary bypass surgery: a prospective randomized study. Br J Haematol 1989;72:81-4.
112. AABB makes recommendations regarding directed donations and graft-versus-host disease. News Briefs 1989; 12:1-2.

In: Kurtz SR, Baldwin ML and Sirchia G, eds.
Controversies in Transfusion Medicine:
Immune Complications and Cytomegalovirus Transmission
Arlington, VA: American Association
of Blood Banks, 1990

5

Cytomegalovirus Infection in Clinical Transplantation: The Role of Transfusion Support Using Donors Seronegative for Cytomegalovirus

Hayden G. Braine, MD

C YTOMEGALOVIRUS (CMV) IS A ubiquitous pathogen generally causing minimal morbidity in the healthy host. In the immune-compromised patient, however, the consequences of CMV infection can carry not only significant morbidity, but also mortality.

CMV was not successfully cultured in vitro until 1956. However, because of its unique large cytoplasmic inclusions, disease related to what was subsequently identified as CMV had been recognized for over 100 years. First described in 1889, these pathoneumonic inclusions were first observed in the kidneys of congenitally infected infants. Subsequently, congenital CMV infection has been associated with a variety of developmental defects of the central nervous system.[1,2]

It was not until 1965 that it was appreciated that CMV was the agent responsible for endemic heterophile negative mononucleosis. During this period CMV infection was also recognized as a side effect of blood transfusion. It was the practice to use fresh whole blood in open-heart surgery. A "post-pump" syndrome characterized by fever, hepatitis and prolonged malaise was commonly encountered. In 1966, Kaariainen recog-

---

Hayden G. Braine, MD, Associate Professor of Oncology, Johns Hopkins Oncology Center, Baltimore, Maryland

nized that this syndrome was related to transfusion-transmitted CMV infection.[3] Subsequently, a similar posttransfusion syndrome was described in neonates. Whereas adult CMV-related mononucleosis was generally not fatal, this was not the case in neonatal infections. However, disseminated CMV infection in severely immunosuppressed adults is also associated with a high mortality. This was initially appreciated in recipients of renal and bone marrow transplants, but has also been described following liver and cardiac transplantation.

To date, there has been some degree of fatalism about CMV infections. This is because, in general, the consequences of these infections have been mild, and the ubiquitous nature of the agent would seem to mitigate against its effective control. However, CMV can have devastating effects during intrauterine differentiation and in conjunction with severe immunosuppression. Current technology offers the ability to abolish at least one route of transmission. However, the routine production of blood components free of CMV infectivity is costly and logistically difficult. Furthermore, it is not clear that all patients will benefit from CMV-negative transfusion support. This chapter explores the appropriate role of CMV-negative blood transfusion in the transplant patient.

Molecular Biology of the Cytomegalovirus

CMV is the largest virus of the herpes family. This family includes Herpes simplex viruses (types I and II), Herpes zoster (varicella), the Epstein-Barr virus and CMV itself. As a group these viruses are characterized structurally by a core of double-stranded DNA surrounded by a complex capsid structure. Biologically, they are characterized by latency in the infected host.

Following infection with the CMV agent, cells undergo a sequence of molecular events. The earliest is characterized by the appearance in the cell membrane of an immediate early protein (IE) with a molecular weight of approximately 68,000. This protein is followed by a sequence of eight additional early proteins (EA).[4,5] These early proteins are clinically important as they represent characteristic cell surface markers of infected cells. Monoclonal antibodies to these proteins can be used to detect CMV in infected tissues.

Early in the course of infection, CMV DNA becomes incorporated into the host's DNA. This results in a latent state during which there is no evidence of free virus, and yet CMV DNA can be detected in the genome using molecular hybridization techniques. During infection with CMV, the host sequentially produces IgM and IgG antibodies. Despite the presence of these antibodies, CMV infection apparently can continue to spread in the host by direct cell-to-cell transmission or by overwhelming viremia.

During active infection with herpes viruses, multiple tissues are infected. However, latency capable of producing reactivation of infection apparently is characteristic of a limited number of tissues. The Herpes simplex viruses are dormant in sensory neurons of the oral and genital mucous membranes, whereas Herpes zoster infects ganglions of cutaneous sensory nerves. Reactivation of these viruses is clinically recognized as "cold sores" or "shingles."

The host cell for latent CMV infection has not been definitively demonstrated. Multiple investigators have shown persistence of the DNA genome with the presence of IE and/or EA antigens in cells of both the granulocyte and monocyte lineage.[5-7] Other investigators have demonstrated convincing evidence that the T cell may also be a host of latent CMV. Clinically, these observations are important as they apparently account for the ease with which CMV infection can be transmitted by transfusions containing cellular elements. As currently prepared, all cellular components (red cells, platelets and, of course, granulocytes) are heavily contaminated with leukocytes. If truly leukocyte-free components could be manufactured, it is conceivable that DNA-free red cells and platelet concentrates should be free of the risk of transmitting CMV infection.

Multiple factors can reactivate latent herpes viruses. These include emotional as well as physical/chemical factors. In the case of the cytomegalovirus, spontaneous reactivation of infection due to emotional or physical stress is not well-recognized. The creation of deficits in the host's immune surveillance, however, can be an important trigger of latent infection. In this regard, transfusion itself may be an important trigger of latent CMV infection.[5,6]

It is now clear that blood transfusion results in some degree of immunosuppression. Following blood transfusion, a variety of changes take place in various cellular subsets of the immune system. These include changes in NK cells, suppressor cell activity and helper cell activity.[5,6] Reactivation of latent CMV may be a consequence of such posttransfusion immunosuppression. Thus, transfusion itself may paradoxically be a major factor in determining the development of posttransfusion CMV infection. This may account for the fact that the risk of developing CMV infection from blood components is not linear: The risk of infection becomes disproportionately higher the larger the number of units transfused.

Spectrum of Disease Caused by CMV

The clinical manifestations of CMV infection are highly variable depending on patient susceptibility (Table 5-1). Infection in the immune-competent host is usually asymptomatic. However, in the fetus or immunosuppressed host, CMV infection can be devastating.

Serologically, three types of CMV infection can be recognized: primary infection, reactivation of latent infection and reinfection. Primary infection occurs in the seronegative host and is generally more symptomatic in the recipient of a solid organ transplant than secondary infection. Secondary infections are either reactivation of a latent primary infection or acquisition of an immunologically distinctive new strain of CMV. Although reinfection appears to be rare, it has been shown to occur in renal transplant patients.[8]

Congenital infection with CMV has been associated with a characteristic syndrome termed cytomegalic inclusion disease (CID). CID is recognized as the cause of a spectrum of birth defects including neuromuscular deficits such as microcephaly, intracerebral calcifications, chorioretinitis and motor disabilities. This syndrome is perhaps one of the least commented upon aspects of the public health impact of CMV infection and the least considered when prophylaxis of CMV infection is discussed.

CMV infection can likewise be devastating in low-birth-weight neonates. In the 1970's, Ballard first reported a syndrome of respiratory deterioration, hepatosplenomegaly and lymphocytosis in low-birth-weight infants. Subsequent studies implicated the CMV agent in this frequently fatal disease. It was further identified that blood transfusion was the principle route of infection.[5,6]

In the immune-competent adult, CMV has a much milder course and is usually characterized as a heterophile negative mononucleosis syndrome. The symptom complex involves fever, pharyngitis, generalized lymphadenopathy and lymphocytosis. To a lesser degree, hepatitis is also characteristic of this syndrome. Most primary CMV infections in the immune-competent host are asymptomatic.

Table 5-1. Clinical Manifestations of CMV Infection

I. *Cytomegalic Inclusion Disease (CID)*
— Jaundice hepatosplenomegaly, petechiae
— Neuromuscular deficits
    — microcephaly
    — cerebral calcification
    — chorioretinitis
    — motor disabilities
— asymptomatic retardation
    — low IQ
    — school failure
    — hearing loss

II. *Heterophile Negative Mononucleosis*
— hepatitis
— lymphadenopathy/lymphocytosis
— fever
— pharyngitis
— uncommon syndromes
    — interstitial pneumonitis
    — inflammatory polyneuropathy
    — meningoencephalitis
    — thrombocytopenia
    — hemolytic anemia

III. *Disseminated CMV Infection in Immune-Compromised Host*
— asymptomatic
— mononucleosis
— interstitial pneumonitis
— retinitis
— arthritis
— opportunistic infection
    — fungus
    — bacteria
    — pneumocystis
— colitis/gastritis
— vesicular skin rash
— interstitial nephritis/hematuria
— glomerulonephritis
— GVHD or organ rejection

CMV infection in the immune-compromised host, however, can be serious. A mononucleosis-like syndrome with or without viremia is not uncommon. In addition, retinitis, colitis and gastritis have been reported. Hematological abnormalities include leukocytosis, thrombocytopenia and hemolytic anemia. Sporadic cases of myocarditis, meningeal encephalitis and acute Guillain-Barré syndrome have also been reported. Tubular nephritis and immune complex glomerulonephritis have been noted in association with CMV infection (Table 5-1).

Epidemiology of CMV Infection

Endemic CMV infection is usually transmitted by close contact. The prevalence of CMV infection increases with age, lower socioeconomic status and possibly residence in northern latitudes.[5,6] Women are more likely to have had prior CMV infection, perhaps related to child care. These factors account for a wide variability in the incidence of CMV seropositivity in various populations. In some third world populations, CMV infection may approach 100%. In other populations it may be as low as 40%. In most regions of the United States, the incidence of CMV seropositivity has run between 40% and 60%.[5,6]

Blood and body fluids have been implicated in transmission of CMV infection. The virus has been detected in saliva, urine and breast milk. Blood and organ transplants can also transmit infection. Epidemiologic studies have reported the risk of CMV infection for immunosuppressed patients to be from 3-12% per unit of cellular components transfused. The risk of CMV transmission with cellular blood components to nonimmunosuppressed patients has been reported to be as low as 0.1% to 0.4%.[9] On the basis of current understanding of blood-transmitted CMV infection, the following can be stated:

1. CMV-seropositive blood components containing cellular elements transmit CMV infection.
2. The infectivity rate is low; not all seropositive units will transmit CMV.
3. The incidence of CMV infection will depend on the following:
   a. the number of units transfused;
   b. the type of blood component. (eg, frozen deglycerolized red cells have essentially no risk whereas the risk from granulocyte transfusion is high);
   c. the susceptibility of the patient (imunosuppressed patients have a higher incidence of infection).

Patterns of Infection Following Organ Transplantation

Allogeneic Bone Marrow Transplantation (BMT)

Historically, CMV infection has been one of the leading causes of morbidity and mortality in patients undergoing allogeneic bone marrow transplantation. In a recent review of 521 patients undergoing allogeneic BMT at the Johns Hopkins Oncology Center, overall 46% of patients developed evidence of CMV infection.[10] Viremia was detected in 12% of cases, a median of 44 days after transplant. Seroconversion was more common, occurring in 37% of the cases, at a mean of 55 days post-transplant. In most cases, CMV infection was subclinical. Clinical symptoms, when present, were variable. The most common syndrome was fever of unknown etiology with or without associated arthralgia and/or myalgia. Abnormal liver functions in this context were frequently observed, but their etiology was usually multifactional. A small number of patients manifested enterocolitis and a few retinitis.[10,11]

By far the most serious complication of CMV infection during bone marrow transplantation has been interstitial pneumonitis. This syndrome is characterized by the development of bilateral nonlobar pulmonary infiltrates with associated dyspnea, tachypnea and hypoxia. To attribute this syndrome to CMV, characteristic intranuclear inclusions need to be demonstrated histopathologically or CMV itself cultured from lung tissue. In nearly all published series, CMV has been the most commonly documented cause of interstitial pneumonitis following bone marrow transplantation. In our experience at Hopkins, CMV has accounted for 8% of all the cases of interstitial pneumonitis in which an infectious agent could be demonstrated. Of critical importance is the fact that once diagnosed, CMV pneumonitis is fatal in over 80% of patients who develop it.[11] It should be noted that in recent years there has been a dramatic decrease in CMV-related interstitial pneumonitis following BMT. This decrease may relate to the use of acyclovir as prophylaxis for Herpes simplex infection, use of CMV-seronegative blood support, more effective therapy or other factors.

Several large studies have identified risks factors associated with CMV interstitial pneumonitis.[12-15] These include treatment for hematological malignancies, older age, use of granulocyte transfusions, acute graft-vs-host disease and duration and type of immunosuppression. Seropositive allograft recipients were at greater risk for developing interstitial pneumonitis than were seronegative allograft recipients receiving grafts from seropositive donors.

In the 1970's, most major centers performing bone marrow transplants employed either therapeutic or prophylactic strategies for granulocyte transfusions. An analysis of this practice reveals that recipients of granulocyte transfusion had an untoward incidence of CMV interstitial pneumonitis.[16] Retrospectively, this association would seem obvious as current data would indicate that granulocytes and monocytes, the major cellular fraction of granulocyte transfusions, are the most important cell in transmitting transfusion-related CMV infection. Today, granulocyte transfusions are rarely employed in allogeneic bone marrow transplantation.

In all reported series, there has been a strong association between CMV infection and the development of graft-vs-host disease (GVHD).[14,15] This syndrome is mediated by committed T cells present in the marrow graft, which recognize mismatched transplantation antigens in the patient. The resultant syndrome is characterized by severe dermatitis, hepatitis and enterocolitis. Its management entails the use of various immunosuppressive technologies including prednisone therapy, polyclonal or monoclonal anti-T-cell antibodies and/or cyclosporin A. Over half of the patients developing severe GVHD will die either of GVHD or of a complication related to the concomitant immunosuppression required for the management of the disease. Therefore, one would presume that the association of CMV interstitial pneumonitis with GVHD would be a logical consequence of systemic immunosuppression. However, closer analysis of interstitial pneumonitis in the allogeneic transplant setting indicates that this syndrome may not be entirely caused by direct infection of lung parenchymal tissue with the virus. In fact, there is some evidence that suggests that autoimmune mechanisms may be important in the development of CMV-associated interstitial pneumonitis.[11,17]

This is suggested by two clinical observations. First, there is not a simple relationship between culture-positive CMV infection and interstitial pneumonitis. In fact, CMV may be cultured from the lung at times when no pneumonitis is diagnosed clinically. Second, CMV pneumonitis has proven refractory to treatment with traditional antiviral approaches such as the use of hyperimmune globulin or antiviral chemotherapy. The only reported therapy felt to be effective for CMV-associated interstitial pneumonitis is a combination treatment with high-dose gamma globulin and gancyclovir.[18] It is known that high dose gamma globulin therapy can result in reticuloendothelial blockade. It would be interesting to speculate that the mechanism of action of this therapeutic approach to CMV interstitial pneumonitis may not be through a simple viricidal mechanism, but rather through reticuloendothelial blockade. In any case, these observations suggest that factors other than simple virus load may be involved in CMV interstitial pneumonitis.

The hypothesis that CMV interstitial pneumonitis has an autoimmune component has also been suggested in three mouse models.[17] In summary, these animal data have shown a lack of correlation between pulmonary viral replication and development of interstitial pneumonitis. Further, interstitial pneumonitis was shown to be dependent upon retention of some degree of immune responsiveness on the part of the host. Thus, the animal models strongly suggest a role for host immunity in CMV interstitial pneumonitis.

It has also been observed that CMV infection, either directly or indirectly, can result in an enhanced expression of antigens of the major histocompatibility complex on host cells. This may be due to some interaction of viral proteins with host cell membranes, or perhaps to the action of intermediary lymphokines such as interferon.[17] In any case, it would appear that CMV infections can enhance the expression of histocompatibility antigens and tissues.

Taken together, these data would suggest that CMV interstitial pneumonitis may, in fact, be a component of autoimmune or graft-vs-host disease related to increased antigenic expression of transplantation antigens. This mechanism may also be important in explaining the increased incidence of graft rejection noted following renal transplantation.[19] In any case, if such a mechanism is present, its clinical importance would be quite significant as the therapeutic approach to an immune type pneumonitis may more appropriately be pursued with immunosuppressive therapy rather than with direct antiviral therapy.[17]

Finally, patients undergoing allogeneic bone marrow transplantation without evidence of CMV infection have a faster immunological recovery than those who do manifest CMV infection. Deficits in lymphocyte response to concanavalin A, phytohemagglutinin, anti-β_2-microglobulin and staphylococcal protein A have been noted.[20,21] These deficits seem to be a direct effect of CMV infection.

Autologous Bone Marrow Transplantation

A recent analysis of marrow transplants at Johns Hopkins has indicated that there is no difference between the overall incidence of CMV infection following autologous or allogeneic bone marrow transplantation (Table 5-2).[10] Approximately half of the patients undergoing autologous transplant manifested a CMV infection either by a fourfold rise in anti-CMV antibody titers or by culturing of the virus. However, in the autologous setting, only one patient developed CMV pneumonitis as compared to an incidence of approximately 10% in the allogeneic group. As previously noted, this difference was closely associated with the development of graft-vs-host disease.

Delayed platelet recovery has also been reported following CMV infection in the autologous bone marrow transplant. Verdonck et al[22] have examined the effect of CMV serological status prior to transplant on hematological reconstitution. CMV seronegative transplant patients achieved $5 \times 10^9/L$ (50,000/mm^3) platelets in a mean of 21.5 days posttransplant. This was significantly faster than those patients who were CMV-positive at the time of transplant and did not reach greater than $5 \times 10^9/L$ (50,000/mm^3) platelets until some 40 days after transplant.[22] These observations have been confirmed by Wingard et al in the Hopkins transplant experience.[10] In this series of patients undergoing autologous bone marrow transplant, recovery of the platelet count to $5 \times 10^9/L$ (50,000/mm^3) was markedly delayed in the seropositive group (97 days) vs the seronegative group (25 days). Neutrophil recovery to 500 mL cells was also slower in the seropositive group (31 days vs 24 days).

Fortunately, CMV infection in the autologous bone marrow transplant is associated with less mortality than that observed in the allogeneic setting. Whereas infection is common, fatal interstitial pneumonitis is rare.[14] However, the morbidity associated with delayed hematologic constitution should not be minimized. Prolonged antibiotic and transfusion support re-

Table 5-2. CMV Infection Following Bone Marrow Transplantation: The Johns Hopkins Experience

	Autologous	Allogeneic	p
Number	264	521	
Mean age	22	23	N.S.
CMV infection	49%	46%	N.S.
Primary infection in patients at risk	45%	37%	N.S.
Viremia	3%	12%	<0.0005
Virus excretion	14%	29%	<0.0002
CMV disease	2%	10%	<0.0001

Adapted from Wingard et al.[10]

quired by slow marrow reconstitution has significant economic and medical consequences. If these infections could be avoided, one would anticipate a significant improvement in the posttransplant course of many patients.

Renal Transplants

Sixty to seventy percent of renal transplant candidates are CMV seropositive.[23] With this high incidence of CMV seropositivity in renal transplant recipients, it is not surprising that CMV infection is a major cause of morbidity and mortality following renal transplantation. Posttransplant infection rates have been reported as high as 60-80%.[23] A national strategy to maintain potential transplant recipients on CMV-seronegative blood components could decrease CMV seropositivity among this group of patients.

Numerous studies have documented three important sources of CMV infection in the kidney transplant patient: 1) latent virus in the patient due to prior infection, 2) latent virus in the kidney graft and 3) latent virus in blood transfusion.

This is well-demonstrated in a series of 1245 patients from 46 transplant centers reported by Rubin et al.[19] In this series the critical role of the CMV status of the renal graft was again demonstrated. Eight-two percent of seronegative recipients who received grafts from seropositive donors seroconverted to CMV! This compares to a conversion rate of only 17% in seronegative recipients of seronegative kidneys. Further, in seronegative recipients of seronegative grafts who received only seronegative blood transfusion, there were no seroconversions. Thus, the renal graft and blood transfusion transmit CMV.

The high rate of infection of seronegative recipients receiving seropositive organs is in contrast to the low rate of infectivity from transfused blood. Seronegative transplant recipients receiving transfusion from seropositive blood donors manifested an infection rate of approximately 1 in 20. Thus, the transplanted kidney is some 20 times more infectious than a transfusion of red cells. The reason for this is not clear.

The consequences of CMV infection in the post-kidney-transplant setting is consistent with that following bone marrow transplantation. Serological or microbiological evidence of CMV infection is usually associated with a fever and symptoms of a heterophile negative mononucleosis. Abnormal liver function tests are not uncommon. As in bone marrow transplantation, interstitial pneumonitis associated with CMV infection is the most common cause of mortality. In contrast to the BMT situation, a primary CMV infection in the renal transplant patient has been more symptomatic.[13]

In addition to being a direct cause of infection, CMV infection after renal transplantation has been shown to be associated with an increased incidence of bacterial and fungal super-infections. In one series of 35 renal allograft recipients, of six initially seronegative patients who developed CMV infection, four died of fungal infections. This compared to only one nonfatal fungal infection in 22 seropositive patients.[23] The reason for this has not been definitively demonstrated, but it appears to be related to a global immunosuppression associated with CMV infection.

CMV infection after kidney transplantation has also been associated with an increased incidence of organ rejection. In one multicenter trial, the effect of CMV on organ rejection was most significant in patients receiving antithymocyte globulin and undergoing a primary CMV infection: 71% graft retention at 6 months was noted for patients with secondary infections vs 53% for those with primary infections.[19] Again, the reason for this has not been proven, but the associated increase in membrane expression of histocompatibility antigens during CMV infection may account for this phenomenon. The increased incidence of organ rejection following renal transplantation may be analogous to the increased incidence of graft-vs-host disease following bone marrow transplantation.

Finally, CMV infection has been associated with an increased incidence of membranous glomerulonephropathy in the posttransplant setting. This may be an additional cause of renal graft failure in the CMV-infected patient.

Many kidney transplant centers administer leukocyte transfusions pretransplant to increase graft survival. The immunologic reason for this improvement remains unknown. When living related donors (LRD) are used, the kidney donor may also be the leukocyte donor. When unrelated grafts are used, leukocyte transfusions are usually pooled leukocytes from random donors (RD). Chou et al have examined the effect of such transfusion on CMV seropositivity.[24] In a series of 76 seronegative kidney transplants, Chou examined the effect of transfusion of approximately 2×10^9 irradiated cells from CMV-seropositive donors. Donors of LRD leukocytes were known to be CMV-seropositive. RD leukocyte transfusion contained cells from five donors. Assuming a seropositivity rate of 45%, one could be 99% sure at least one of these five transfusions came from a CMV-seropositive donor. Thus, all RD and LRD were given at least one transfusion from a CMV-seropositive donor.

Table 5-3. Seroconversion Following Pre-Renal Transplant Leukocyte Transfusion

Source of Leukocytes	Number of Transfusions/Donors	Pretransplant CMV Seroconversion Number/Total	(%)
Related kidney donor (LRD)	2/1*	3/8	(38%)
Nonrelated pool (RD)	2/5†	1/32	(3%)

Adapted from Chou et al.[24]
*Known to be CMV seropositive
†99% Certain to contain at least one CMV seropositive donor

All recipients were followed for CMV seroconversion for at least 6 weeks prior to transplant. (See Table 5-3.)

Surprisingly, only 1 of 32 (3%) recipients of RD leukocytes seroconverted, whereas 3 of 5 (38%) recipients of LRD did so. The reason for these observations remains unclear. These data suggest that concern over CMV seroconversion need not absolutely contraindicate pretransplant leukocyte transfusion from RD. CMV seropositive LRD donors, however, should probably be used with caution.

As previously mentioned, use of CMV-seronegative blood in seronegative recipients of seronegative organs eliminates CMV infection. Seronegative patients receiving organs from seropositive donors clearly acquire CMV from the organ graft. On the other hand, it is equally clear that seronegative recipients receiving organs from seronegative donors receive their exposure through seropositive blood transfusion. Thus, seronegative recipients of seronegative organs should be transfused with only CMV-negative blood.

The use of CMV-seronegative blood in CMV-seropositive recipients or with CMV-seropositive organs remains more problematic. Most data suggest the majority of CMV infections in this setting are reactivation of latent virus. Reinfection with a new virus has been demonstrated in seropositive patients.[25] Additional studies will be required to determine if there may be a role for the use of seronegative blood components in seropositive transplant recipients.

Table 5-4. Incidence of CMV and Other Opportunistic Infection After Solid Organ Transplantation

| | Type of Transplant | | |
	Renal	Cardiac	Liver
Number	64	17	24
Mean age	34	40	35
% of patients infected posttransplant (nonviral)	41%	53%	67%
% CMV infection:			
A) Pretransplant CMV seropositive	80%	100%	70%
B) Pretransplant CMV seronegative	44%	100%	62%
C) Total	75%	100%	66%

Modified from Dummer JS, Hardy A, Poorsattar A, Ho M. Early infections in kidney, heart, and liver transplant recipients on cyclosporine. Transplantation 1983;36,3:259-67.

Cardiac and Liver Transplants

Experience today with cardiac and liver transplants is in general consistent with that experienced in renal transplant (Table 5-4). Most infections are asymptomatic. CMV hepatitis, mononucleosis and pneumonitis are not uncommon. In cardiac transplantation, CMV infection has also been associated with an increased rate of nonviral opportunistic infection.[26,27] The donor heart has also been implicated as the source of CMV infection when CMV-seronegative blood has been used. Similar observations have been made following liver transplantation.[28,29] In cardiac and liver transplantation, CMV infection is an important cause of morbidity and mortality. In seronegative recipients of seronegative organs, this can be prevented with seronegative blood transfusion.[26,28]

However, in these clinical settings, maintaining the seronegative status of organ recipients is often difficult. There is a clinically significant organ shortage such that selection of seronegative organs for seronegative recipients is generally not feasible. Further, transfusion support required during the transplant surgery itself is much more extensive than that needed in renal transplants. A significant number of patients undergoing renal transplant may in fact require no transfusion for the surgical procedure itself. On the other hand, it is not uncommon for patients undergoing liver transplant to use 50 different blood components on an emergency basis.[30] For these reasons, it has been difficult to protect many seronegative organ recipients from CMV infection.

Approaches to Prevention of Posttransfusion CMV Infection

CMV-Seronegative Blood Support

Pilot studies indicate that if CMV-seronegative recipients of CMV-seronegative organs are supported with CMV-seronegative blood transfusions, CMV infection can be eliminated. This has been shown in bone marrow,[31-34] renal,[19] cardiac[27] and liver[29,35] transplantation. All reported series of CMV-seronegative transfusion for CMV-seronegative organ/recipient pairs have been nearly 100% effective in preventing CMV infection. Experience in prevention of transfusion-related CMV infection in neonates using CMV screened blood has also been highly effective. (See subsequent chapters.)

The critical question is not: "Is selective transfusion support effective?" The questions are: "Is it necessary?" and "Is it feasible?"

Is It Necessary?

CMV is a major cause of morbidity and mortality following transplantation. To date, attempts to treat infections have not been successful. Newer agents such as foscarnet (trisodium phosphonoformate hexahydrate)[36,37] and gancyclovir [9-(1,3-dihydroxy-2-propoxymethyl) guanine][38,39] have shown some promise, but have not yet been shown to be reliably effective. As previously noted, combination therapy with gancyclovir and immunoglobulin has also shown some promise.[18] Nonetheless, at this time, no proven agent is available to manage established CMV infection or to allow effective prophylaxis.

Attempts at prophylaxis of infection with hyperimmune globulin or gammaglobulin have been somewhat more effective. Summarizing five controlled studies, Sullivan has noted an overall reduction of CMV infections from 43% to 30% using immunoglobulin prophylaxis.[40] While this represents a significant clinical effect, the failure to achieve 100% prophylaxis means it has little applicability in prevention of transfusion-related CMV infection in seronegative transplant patients. Alternatives to CMV-seronegative transfusion support must be as effective as CMV-seronegative transfusion, ie, 100% effective. Currently there is no effective alternative to CMV-sero-negative support in the seronegative recipient of a seronegative graft.

Is It Feasible?

At this time, there is no definitive test available to indicate which CMV-seropositive donors are at risk to transmit CMV infection. It is clear that not all donors who have had prior CMV infection (as evidenced by CMV seropositivity) are infectious. Determination of the noninfectious status of seropositive blood donors would be a significant boon to the prevention of CMV infection as, in most donor centers, only 40-60% of donors test negative for prior infection with CMV. Some authors have suggested that evidence of IgM seroconversion has a stronger correlation with infectivity than IgG seroconversion. Definitive proof of this hypothesis, however, is pending.

Selection of a testing methodology of sufficient sensitivity for CMV screening was initially considered a major impediment to donor screening. However, today there are several FDA-approved kits capable of sufficient sensitivity, economy and speed to be practical for screening large populations of blood donors. At Johns Hopkins we use a sensitive latex agglutination technology. Donors are not considered seronegative until they have been tested on two separate occasions and found to be sero-negative. They are then retested at the time of each donation.

Maintenance of supplies of CMV-negative red cells is made easier due to the long shelf life of red cells. When CMV-negative red cells are needed for specific cases, inventories of ABO-specific CMV-negative blood can be reserved for specific patient use. In situations where platelet transfusions are required, logistics are more complex. However, most facilities that have access to a plateletpheresis program can arrange for prospective donation of sufficient platelet products to support the CMV-seronegative patient through aplasia. The extension of platelet storage to 5 days also has been most helpful in this regard.[30] Selected blood centers can also supply CMV-sero-negative pooled multiple donor concentrates.

A final complexity of development of a CMV-negative blood program has not been closely examined. While preferential diversion of CMV-seronegative blood resources to CMV-sero-negative recipients has a logical basis, operationally this results in an increased possibility that other patients will receive CMV-seropositive blood transfusions. Thus, many CMV-seronegative or CMV-seropositive nontransplant patients will receive seropositive blood. While there is no clear case for increased mortality associated with such policies, it would seem to have the potential for some increase in morbidity. Whenever CMV-negative blood programs are instituted, consideration of such reverse triage of CMV-seropositive blood components should be carefully evaluated.

Who Will Benefit From CMV-Seronegative Blood Support?

Clearly, CMV-seronegative recipients of CMV-seronegative bone marrow, kidney, cardiac and liver transplant will benefit. By extension, CMV-seronegative candidates for organ transplantation should also be maintained with CMV-seronegative transfusion.

Management of the CMV-seropositive recipient or the CMV-seronegative recipient of a CMV-seropositive organ is more problematic. In this setting the incidence of true reinfection is presumed to be low. In fact, the true rate of reinfection from transfusion is not known. At this time, CMV seronegative support for this group should be undertaken only in the context of a clinical trial.

Future Directions

CMV-seronegative organ transplant recipients receiving grafts from seronegative donors clearly benefit from the preferential use of CMV-negative blood support. Although development of a seronegative blood support program is difficult, it can be achieved at most major centers supporting organ transplantation. However, if this service is to be more generally applicable, the availability of CMV-negative or noninfectious blood will have to be increased. As previously discussed, the possibility of identifying markers for infectivity such as IgM anti-CMV titers could significantly increase the number of noninfectious donors. It would appear that CMV is being transmitted in the posttransfusion situation via donor leukocytes (granulocytes, monocytes, T cells). Platelets and red cells lacking nuclei (and, therefore, DNA) should theoretically be free of risk of transmitting CMV. Unfortunately, currently available red cell and platelet concentrates contain a significant number of leukocytes capable of transmitting CMV. Removal of leukocytes from these products may render them free of risk of transmitting CMV. In order to be effective, leukocyte depletion may need to be complete. Two log reductions (99%) in white cells are probably inadequate.

Initial data indicated that "washed" red cells may have reduced risk for CMV transmission.[41] Unfortunately, this has not been borne out in additional studies. Red cells prepared by freezing and deglycerolization have a significantly reduced risk of transmitting CMV.[42,43] Apparently, the leukocyte loss incurred by freeze-thaw damage combined with vigorous "washing" is sufficient to prevent CMV transmission. Frozen de-glycerolized red cells are expensive and logistically difficult to obtain. Alternate techniques for leukodepletion would be pref-erable.

Newer "fourth generation" filters such as the Pall RC-100,® PL-100® (Pall Corporation, Glen Cove, NY) and others are reported to reduce leukocyte contamination to 10^4 to 10^6 cells per transfusion.[44] This degree of depletion may be sufficient to eliminate the risk of CMV transmission. In one early series reported in abstract, 0/20 bone marrow patients receiving leukocyte-poor blood components developed CMV infection, whereas 7/25 in the control group did so.[45] Further experience will be required to confirm this important finding.

Summary

CMV infection causes significant morbidity and mortality in the immune-compromised patient. CMV infection may exert its adverse effects through direct cellular toxicity, through its suppressive effect on the immune system or by regulating histocompatibility antigens with resultant worsening of GVHD or graft rejection.

In the posttransplant situation, CMV infection may be a primary or reinfection transmitted by transfusion or the graft itself. In other cases, it may represent reactivation of latent infection. At this time, there is no reliable therapy for estab-lished infection. Hence, management must focus on prevention of primary infection in the CMV-seronegative transplant pa-tient. All potential CMV-seronegative transplant recipients should be maintained on CMV-seronegative transfusion sup-port until transplant. If a seronegative organ can be obtained, CMV-seronegative transfusion should be continued.

Acknowledgments

The author is indebted to Cindy Young and Beverly Davis for expert assistance in manuscript preparation.

References

1. Weller TH. The cytomegaloviruses: Ubiquitous agents with protean clinical manifestations (First of Two Parts). N Engl J Med 1971;285:203-14.
2. Weller TH. The cytomegaloviruses: Ubiquitous agents with protean clinical manifestations (Second of Two Parts). N Engl J Med 1971;285:267-74.
3. Kaariainen L, Paloheimo J, Klemola E, et al. Cytomegalovirus-mononucleosis: Isolation of the virus and demonstration of subclinical infections after fresh blood transfusion in connection with open-heart surgery. Ann Med Exp Biol Fenn 1966;44:297-301.
4. Adler SP. Transfusion-associated cytomegalovirus infections. Infect Dis 1983;5:977-93.
5. Tegtmeier GE. Transfusion-transmitted cytomegalovirus infections: Significance and control. Vox Sang 1986;51:22-30.
6. Einhorn L, Ost A. Cytomegalovirus infection of human blood cells. J Infect Dis 1984;149:207-14.
7. Tegtmeier GE. Cytomegalovirus infection as a complication of blood transfusion. Semin Liv Dis 1986;6:82-95.
8. Adler SP. Cytomegalovirus and transfusions. Transf Med Rev 1988;2:235-44.
9. Preiksaitis JK, Brown L, McKenzie M. The risk of cytomegalovirus infections in seronegative transfusion recipients not receiving exogenous immunosuppression. J Infect Dis 1988;157:523-9.
10. Wingard JR, Chen DYH, Burns WH, et al. Cytomegalovirus infection after autologous bone marrow transplantation with comparison to infection after allogeneic bone marrow transplantation. Blood 1988;71:1432-7.
11. Zaia JA. The biology of human cytomegalovirus infection after bone marrow transplantation. Int J Cell Cloning 1086;4:135-54.
12. Paulin T, Ringden O, Lonnqvist B, et al. The importance of pre bone marrow transplantation serology in determining subsequent cytomegalovirus infection: An analysis of risk factors. Scand J Infect Dis 1986;18:199-209.
13. Guyotat D, Gibert R, Chomel J, et al. Incidence and prognosis of cytomegalovirus infections following allogenic bone marrow transplantation. J Med Virol 1987;23:393-9.
14. Wingard JR, Sostrin MB, Vriesendorp HM, et al. Interstitial pneumonitis following autologous bone marrow transplantation. Transplantation 1988;46:61-5.

15. Lonnqvist B, Ringden O, Wahren B, et al. Cytomegalovirus infection associated with and preceding chronic graft-versus-host-disease. Transplantation 1984;38:465-8.
16. Winston DJ, Ho WG, Howell CL, et al. Cytomegalovirus infections associated with leukocyte transfusions. Ann Intern Med 1980;93:671-5.
17. Grundy JE, Shanley JD, Griffiths PD. Is cytomegalovirus interstitial pneumonitis in transplant recipients an immunopathological condition? Lancet 1987;2:996-9.
18. Reed EC, Bowden RA, Dandliker PS, et al. Treatment of cytomegalovirus pneumonia with gancyclovir and intra-venous cytomegalovirus immunoglobulin in patients with bone marrow transplants. Ann Intern Med 1988;783-8.
19. Rubin RH, Tolkoff-Rubin NE, Oliver D, et al. Multicenter seroepidemiologic study of the impact of cytomegalovirus infection on renal transplantation. Transplantation 1985; 40:243-9.
20. Paulin T, Ringden O, Lonnqvist B. Faster immunological recovery after bone marrow transplantation in patients without cytomegalovirus infection. Transplantation 1985; 39:377-84.
21. Verdonck LF, van der Linden JA, Bast BJ, Gmelig Meyling FH. Influence of cytomegalovirus infection on the recovery of humoral immunity after autologous bone marrow transplantation. Exp Hematol 1987;15:864-8.
22. Verdonck LF, van Heugten H, de Gast GC. Delay in platelet recovery after bone marrow transplantation: Impact of cytomegalovirus infection. Blood 1985;66:921-5.
23. Glenn J. Cytomegalovirus infections following renal transplantation. Rev Infect Dis 1981;3:1151-78.
24. Chou S. Transmission of cytomegalovirus by pre-transplant leukocyte transfusions in renal transplant candidates. J Infect Dis 1987;155:565-7.
25. Grundy JE, Super M, Sweny P, et al. Symptomatic cytomegalovirus infection in seropositive kidney recipients: Reinfection with donor virus rather than reactivation of recipient virus. Lancet 1988:1:132-5.
26. Preiksaitis JK, Rosno S, Grumet C, Merigan TC. Infections due to herpesviruses in cardiac transplant recipients: Role of the donor heart and immunosuppressive therapy. J Infect Dis 1983;147:974-81.
27. Pollard RB, Arvin AM, Gamberg P, et al. Specific cell-mediated immunity and infections with herpes viruses in cardiac transplant recipients. Am J Med 1982;73:679-87.
28. Dussaix E, Wood C. Cytomegalovirus infection in pediatric liver recipients. Transplantation 1989;48:272-4.

29. Rakela J, Wiesner RH, Taswell HF, et al. Incidence of cytomegalovirus infection and its relationship to donor-recipient serologic status in liver transplantation. Transplant Proc 1987;14:2399-402.
30. Butler P, Israel L, Nusbacher J, et al. Blood transfusion in liver transplantation. Transfusion 195;25:120-3.
31. Bowden RA, Sayers M, Gleaves CA, et al. Cytomegalovirus-seronegative blood components for the prevention of primary cytomegalovirus infection after marrow transplantation. Considerations for blood banks. Transfusion 1987; 27:478-81.
32. Mahmoud HK, Beelen DW, Neumann MC, et al. Cytomegalovirus hyperimmunoglobulin and substitution with blood products from antibody-negative donors. A pilot study in bone marrow transplant recipients. Hamatol Bluttransfus 1987;30:538-40.
33. Bowden Rh, Sayers M, Flournoy N, et al. Cytomegalovirus immune globulin and seronegative blood products to prevent primary cytomegalovirus infection after bone marrow transplantation. J Engl J Med 1986;314:1006-10.
34. MacKinnon S, Burnett AK, Crawford RJ, et al. Seronegative blood products prevent primary cytomegalovirus infection after bone marrow transplantation. J Clin Pathol 1988;41:948-50.
35. Breinig MK, Zitelli B, Starzl TE, Ho M. Epstein-Barr virus, cytomegalovirus, and other viral infections in children after liver transplantation. J Infect Dis 1987;156:273-9.
36. Klintmalm G, Lonnqvist B, et al. Intravenous foscarnet for the treatment of severe cytomegalovirus infection in allograft recipients. Scand J Infect Dis 1985;17:157-63.
37. Ringden O, Lonnqvist B, Faulin T, et al. Pharmacokinetics, safety and preliminary clinical experiences using foscarnet in the treatment of cytomegalovirus infections in bone marrow and renal transplant recipients. J Antimicrob Chemother 1986;17:373-87.
38. Keay S, Rissett J, Merigan TC. Gancyclovir treatment of cytomegalovirus infections in iatrogenically immuno-compromised patients. J Infect Dis 1987;156:1016-21.
39. Collaborative DHPG Treatment Study Group. Treatment of serious cytomegalovirus infections with 9-(1,3-dihydroxy-2-propoxymcthyl) guanine in patients with AIDS and other immunodeficiencies. N Engl J Med 1986;314:801-5.
40. Sullivan KM. Immunoglobulin therapy in bone marrow transplantation. Am J Med 1987;83:34-45.
41. Luban NLC, Williams AE, MacDonald MG, et al. Low incidence of acquired cytomegalovirus infection in neonates

transfused with washed red blood cells. Am J Dis Child 1987;141:416-9.

42. Taylor BJ, Jacogs RF, Baker RL, et al. Frozen deglycerolyzed blood prevents transfusion-acquired cytomegalovirus infections in neonates. Pediatr Infect Dis 1986; 5:188-91.

43. Tegtmeier GE. The use of cytomegalovirus-screened blood in neonates.Transfusion 1988;28:201-3.

44. Ciavarella D, Snyder E. Clinical use of blood transfusion devices. Transf Med Rev 1988;2:95-111.

45. Bowden RA, Sayers M, Slichter SJ, Meyers JD. Use of leukocyte-poor transfusions to prevent transfusion-associated cytomegalovirus (CMV) infection after marrow transplant (abstract). Second International CMV Workshop, San Diego, March 1989. San Diego: University of California 1989:67.

In: Kurtz SR, Baldwin ML and Sirchia G, eds.
Controversies in Transfusion Medicine:
Immune Complications and Cytomegalovirus Transmission
Arlington, VA: American Association
of Blood Banks,1990

6

Cytomegalovirus-Seronegative Blood Support for Perinatal Patients—CON

Jutta K. Preiksaitis, MD

C YTOMEGALOVIRUS (CMV) IS KNOWN to be transmitted by blood transfusion. However, transfusion-acquired CMV infection differs significantly from most other virus infections transmitted by blood components. Infections such as hepatitis B and C and human immunodeficiency virus (HIV) are believed to result from the transmission of infectious virus present in the blood of chronically and persistently infected donors or donors experiencing a primary infection.[1-3] A relatively small proportion of blood donors are infected with these viruses and extremely good, although imperfect, serological techniques are available for screening and excluding these donors.[1,2,4] In contrast, CMV is believed to be transmitted in a latent, noninfectious state by blood components and is reactivated after transfusion into the recipient.[5-7] As a result, recipient host factors may be as important or, perhaps, more important than donor factors in determining the risk of acquiring CMV infection from blood components.

CMV antibody prevalence rates in industrialized countries including Canada, the United States, Australia and western Europe vary from 30-80%.[5-7] At the present time, all seropositive donors must be considered to have the potential of transmitting CMV. In order to provide CMV-"safe" blood for use in

Jutta K. Preiksaitis, MD, Associate Professor, Department of Medicine, University of Alberta and Consultant, Canadian Red Cross Society Blood Transfusion Service (Edmonton Center), Edmonton, Alberta, Canada

patient populations at high risk of CMV-associated morbidity, cellular blood components from these donors must be excluded or rendered leukocyte-free. As the immunosuppressed populations for whom these blood components are requested increase, considerable stress is placed on blood banks to maintain adequate inventories of these components and determine priorities for the distribution of a limited resource while minimizing the costs associated with the provision of this service. In many populations for whom these components are requested, the morbidity associated with CMV infection is high but the incidence of transfusion-acquired CMV infection has not been clearly documented and the benefit of providing these products has not been proven.[5-7]

The issue is even more confusing in the area of neonatal transfusions where significant differences in both the incidence and morbidity associated with transfusion-acquired CMV infection have been reported.[6,8-13] In centers that have documented a high incidence of transfusion-acquired CMV infection and morbidity in neonates, and have eliminated this risk with the use of CMV-seronegative and leukocyte-free blood components, it would be foolish to suggest that the use of these components is not necessary. However, it is not at all clear why some centers have documented a very low incidence of CMV infection in transfused neonates and whether the use of specialized blood components in these centers is necessary.

We are handicapped in addressing this problem by our lack of understanding of the pathogenesis of transfusion-acquired CMV infection, including knowledge regarding the site of viral latency and factors controlling CMV reactivation. This chapter will review the information available with regard to the incidence of transfusion-acquired CMV infection in the neonatal population, speculate on the pathogenesis of infection in these patients and outline the problems that make it difficult to formulate clear guidelines regarding the need for CMV-"safe" blood for these infants.

The Problem—A Historical Perspective

In the mid-1970's a high incidence of cytomegaloviruria was observed in exchange-transfused infants[14,15] and transfused preterm infants[16-17] in neonatal intensive care units. Full-term neonates born to CMV-seropositive mothers who acquire CMV infection after birth, as a result of exposure to infected genital secretions or breast milk, are usually asymptomatic and do not suffer the long-term consequences of CMV infection that have been observed in infants infected in utero.[18] However, a self-limited syndrome consisting of respiratory deterioration, hepatosplenomegaly, gray pallor and lymphocytosis was described in association with CMV infection in preterm infants.[19] CMV infection was felt to have contributed to the death of some of these infants.[19] Blood transfusion was implicated as the source of infection and the cause of morbidity in these patients.[14-18,20]

This resulted in a number of studies that examined the incidence of transfusion-acquired CMV infection and evaluated programs of intervention.[6,8-13] The results of these studies are summarized in Table 6-1. In the first of these studies Yeager et al[8] examined the potential efficacy of the use of packed red cells from CMV-seronegative donors in the prevention of transfusion-acquired CMV infection in neonates. Infants born to seronegative and seropositive mothers were randomized separately to receive unscreened or seronegative red cells. In infants born to seronegative mothers, she observed no CMV infection in 90 infants who had received only seronegative blood in contrast to an infection rate of 9.2% (10 of 74 infants) who received unscreened blood and had been exposed to one or more seropositive donors. She identified low-birth-weight infants who had been born to CMV-seronegative mothers and who had received at least 50 mL of blood as being at highest risk. Among infants born to seropositive mothers the use of seronegative red cells did not influence the incidence of CMV infection. The presence of passive CMV antibody appeared to protect them against CMV-associated morbidity.

In a study examining the incidence of transfusion-acquired CMV infection, Adler[9] observed similar infection rates and found infection occurred almost exclusively in low-birth-weight infants born to seronegative mothers who had received a large number of donor exposures and a disproportionately large number of CMV-seropositive units. A recent study by Gilbert et al[13] in seronegative infants confirmed these high infection rates and again identified low birth weight and donor exposures as risk factors for infection. The incidence of transfusion-acquired CMV infection in low-birth-weight (<1200-1500 g) infants born to seronegative mothers was similar in these three studies at 31.8%,[8] 24.0%[9] and 31.0%.[13]

However, a number of other recent studies have found significantly lower rates of transfusion-acquired CMV infection in their neonatal population.[6,10-12] Although published only in abstract form, Smith et al[10] and Tegtmeier et al[6,21] examined the incidence of CMV infection in seronegative transfused neonates weighing less than 1500 and 1250 g, respectively. They demonstrated CMV infection in only two of 23 (9.0%)[10]

Table 6-1. Prospective Studies of the Incidence of Transfusion-Acquired Cytomegalovirus Infection in Neonates Born to Seronegative Mothers

Source (year)	CMV Seroprevalence in Blood Donors	Intervention	No. Patients Infected/ No. Patients Studied (percent)	No. Patients Infected/ No. Low-Birth-Weight Neonates Studied (percent)
Yeager et al (1981)	45.3%	random vs CMV seronegative	10/74 (13.5%) 0/90 (0%)	7/22 (31.8%) [<1200g]‡ 0/16 (0%)
Adler et al (1983)	34%	—	7/76* (9.2%)	7/29* (24%) [<1250g]
Smith et al (abstract 1983)	not given	—	—	2/29 (6.9%) [<1500g]
Tegtmeier et al (abstract 1985)	not given	—	—	2/23 (8.7%) [<1250g]
Lamberson et al (1988)	38%	—	7/222 (3.2%)	4/83 (4.8%) [<1500g]
Preiksaitis et al (1988)	42.5%	—	1/126 (0.8%)	1/41 (2.4%) [<1250g]
Gilbert et al (1989)	46%	unfiltered vs filtered	9/42 (21.4%) 0/30 (0%)	9/29 (31.0%) [<1500g] 0/24 (0%)

*Serostatus of one patient was unknown
‡Low birth weight as defined by the authors

and two of 29 (7%)[6,21] of these infants. In a study at our center, only one of 126 transfused seronegative infants developed CMV infection.[12] This infant was one of 41 infants weighing less than 1250 g. Lamberson et al[11] also found evidence of transfusion-acquired CMV infection in only 7 of 222 (3.2%) seronegative infants. Four of these infected infants were among 83 (4.8%) weighing less than 1500 g. A controlled study undertaken in Toronto examining the use of commercially available intra-venous immunoglobulin for the prevention of transfusion-acquired CMV infection in neonates weighing less than 1500 g was aborted because no transfusion-acquired CMV infection was observed in the 31 initial seronegative infants studied (Prober C, personal communication).

The contribution of CMV infection to symptoms in sick premature neonates who often have multisystem dysfunction is difficult to evaluate. The impact of transfusion-acquired CMV infection on morbidity and mortality in these infants is summarized in Table 6-2. In studies documenting a high incidence of infection, not only did a significant proportion of these patients experience CMV-associated morbidity, CMV infection was felt to have contributed to the death of some of these infants.[8,9] Lamberson et al,[11] who documented a low incidence of CMV infection, felt that in one of the infected infants in his study, CMV infection contributed to death. Although the five infants in three studies[6,10,12] that documented a low incidence of transfusion-acquired CMV infection were symptomatic when infected, no deaths could be attributed to CMV infection. In two[8,9] of the three[8,9,11] studies in which infants born to seropositive mothers were also evaluated, no significant morbidity associated with CMV infection was observed in this subgroup. However, clinical deterioration has been documented in a small number of infants born to seropositive mothers concomitant with the onset of CMV shedding by others.[11,22]

In order to evaluate and explain the variable results obtained, it is important to examine what we know regarding the pathogenesis of transfusion-acquired CMV infection.

CMV and the Leukocyte

Since the mid 1960's a large number of epidemiologic studies has provided indirect evidence that blood components can transmit CMV infection.[5-7] However, only recently (with the demonstration of an identical restriction endonuclease pattern

Table 6-2. Morbidity and Mortality in Neonates With Transfusion-Acquired CMV Infection Born to Seronegative Mothers

Source (year)	Morbidity in Infants <1500 g	Morbidity in Infants >1500 g	Mortality* in Infants <1500 g	Mortality in Infants >1500 g
Yeager et al (1981)	5/7† (50%)	0/3 (0%)	4/7 (57.1%)‡	0/3 (0%)
Adler et al (1983)	6/8§ (75%)	0/0 (0%)	3/8 (37.5%)	0/0 (0%)
Smith et al (abstract 1983)	2/2 (100%)	—	0/2 (0%)	—
Tegtmeier et al (abstract 1985)	2/2 (100%)	—	0/2 (0%)	—
Lamberson et al (1988)	2/5 (40%)	0+?2‖/3 (0-66%)	1/5 (20%)	0/3 (0%)‖
Preiksaitis et al (1988)	1/1 (100%)	0/0 (0%)	0/1 (0%)	0/0 (0%)
Gilbert et al (1989)	5/9 (55.6%)	0/0 (0%)	0/9 (0%)	0/0 (0%)

* In author's opinion CMV contributed to death
† No. patients who experienced morbidity/No. patients infected
‡ This subgroup represents infants <1200 g
§ Serostatus of one patient unknown
‖ Contribution of CMV to morbidity difficult to assess

of DNA from CMV isolates from a blood donor and the infected transfused neonate who received his blood) has direct evidence that blood transfusion transmits CMV infection been available.[23] The high incidence of CMV infection associated with granulocyte transfusions[24,25] and the observation that removal of leukocytes from cellular blood components significantly reduces or eliminates the risk of transmitting CMV infections[13] suggest that CMV is transmitted by leukocytes in blood components.

CMV is present in an infectious form in the polymorphonuclear cells and monocytes of the peripheral blood of acutely infected patients.[26-28] It is not certain whether CMV present in polymorphonuclear leukocytes represents virus that has been phagocytosed[27] or whether CMV replicates in these cells or their progenitors.[28] However, aside from a single report in which CMV was isolated from the leukocytes of 2 of 35 (6%) healthy blood donors,[29] cultures of leukocytes from over a thousand other donors in several laboratories failed to isolate CMV.[5-7]

The bulk of evidence suggests that CMV is most often transmitted in a latent form in blood components and is reactivated after transfusion in the recipient. The cell(s) in which CMV is latent is unknown. Peripheral blood leukocytes cannot be productively infected with CMV in vitro, although a subset of T cells and monocytes express immediate-early gene products.[30,31] Attempts to reactivate CMV from the mononuclear cells of CMV-seropositive subjects have been unsuccessful.[32] Schrier et al,[33] using an in situ hybridization technique, found RNA transcripts of CMV immediate-early genes in a small subset of monocytes and predominantly OKT4+ lymphocytes in healthy seropositive adults. CMV DNA was detected in the mononuclear cells of all 20 CMV-seropositive blood donors using a polymerase chain reaction (PCR) amplification technique.[34] This technique also detected CMV DNA in the mononuclear cells of some CMV-seronegative donors.[33]

Whether this indicates that the PCR assay has poor specificity or high sensitivity for the detection of latently infected blood donors remains to be determined. Using immunohistochemistry and a monoclonal antibody to an immediate-early antigen, Toorkey and Carrigan[35] found evidence that CMV may be latent in a number of tissues in CMV-seropositive adults including brain, kidney, spleen, lung and liver. T lymphocytes and macrophages were among the cell types identified as being latently infected. Based on current evidence the T cell and monocyte represent the most likely sites of CMV latency in peripheral blood.

Donor Factors That Influence the Risk of Transfusion-Acquired CMV Infection

It is not known whether blood from all seropositive donors can transmit CMV or whether a subset of infectious seropositive donors can be identified. Recent studies have suggested that blood components from acutely infected donors or donors reactivating endogenous virus, measured by the presence of CMV-specific IgM, may represent a more infectious subset of blood components.[11,35-37] However, not all infected patients in these studies received CMV IgM-positive blood components and a significant proportion of patients who were not infected received CMV IgM-positive units. This may be a reflection of the sensitivity and specificity of currently available IgM assays. Using a sensitive immunoblot method for the detection of CMV-specific IgM, McVoy and Adler[38] found evidence to suggest that CMV reactivation occurs frequently in immunocompetent seropositive individuals and increases with age. This study confirmed the lack of sensitivity of enzyme immunoassay (EIA) methods for the detection of CMV IgM. It is possible that donors who have acute primary CMV infection or reactivation of CMV may be more infectious because they have a low grade of viremia not readily detectable by standard isolation techniques or a significantly larger subset of their leukocytes are latently infected. CMV may also be more readily reactivated from the leukocytes of patients who have recently experienced primary or reactivation infection.

The use of CMV IgM assays may be a useful alternative to the provision of CMV IgG-seronegative blood, particularly in areas of high CMV donor seroprevalence. Although the study by Lamberson et al[11] demonstrated the potential usefulness of this technique for the prevention of transfusion-acquired CMV infection in neonates, the immunofluorescence assay (IFA) technique he used would not be practical for mass screening in blood banks. Further studies are required to determine the sensitivity of currently available assays and the effect of removal of CMV IgM-positive units on the incidence of transfusion-acquired CMV infection before recommending its use.

If viable leukocytes are required for the transmission of CMV, the extent to which a blood component is contaminated by leukocytes would affect its infectivity. Significant variability in the number of leukocytes and lymphocytes between blood components has been demonstrated.[38] This is probably due to differences in white cell counts in donors added to the poor reproducibility of manual technical procedures for separating and recovering blood components. Cellular blood components—packed red cells and platelet concentrates—contain a significant number of leukocytes.[39] A significantly higher proportion of the leukocytes in platelet concentrates are lymphocytes, reflecting the fact that their density gradient region is very close to that of platelets.[38] Whether platelet concen-trates are more likely to transmit CMV than red cell units is unknown. In contrast, plasma components, particularly fresh frozen plasma, contain few viable leukocytes and plasma appears to be a very low risk component with respect to CMV transmission.[8,40] In fact, passive antibody administered in plasma from seropositive donors may protect the recipient from transfusion-acquired CMV infection.[36]

Blood storage also affects leukocyte viability.[41,42] Although early investigators suggested that fresh whole blood was more infectious than stored citrated blood,[43] others have found no association with blood storage and risk.[44-47] However, in two of these studies,[44,45] the data are difficult to interpret because patients seropositive for CMV antibody prior to transfusion who may have been reactivating endogenous recipient virus are included. In a more recent study of seronegative transfusion recipients, Wilhelm et al[48] again found an increased risk of CMV infection in patients who had received fresh, whole blood. Although there is a strong theoretical basis for assuming that blood storage reduces the risk of CMV transmission, this remains unproven.

Recipient Factors That Influence the Risk of Transfusion-Acquired CMV Infection

Significant evidence exists to support the hypothesis that all seropositive blood donors are capable of transmitting CMV and recipient factors are important in determining which patients will reactivate latent virus transmitted by blood transfusion. The very high incidence of CMV infection that has been reported after exchange transfusion in infants[14,15] and granulocyte transfusions[24,25] in man supports this concept. In our study of seronegative transfusion recipients, we observed that the risk/cellular blood unit transfused was not independent of the number of units received.[49] That is, patients who received more than 30 cellular blood component units had a significantly higher risk/unit transfused of acquiring CMV infection than those who had received fewer units. This suggests that recipient factors are important in determining risk and argues against the idea that eliminating a subgroup of "infectious" seropositive donors will prevent transfusion-acquired CMV infection. It also suggests that the epidemiology of transfusion-acquired CMV infection should be determined for each patient population at risk and that extrapolation of risk from one patient group to another may not be valid.

A Model for the Pathogenesis of Transfusion-Acquired CMV Infection

At least three factors may play a role in the pathogenesis of transfusion-acquired CMV infection. First, a minimum volume of seropositive blood may be required to ensure transfer of a sufficient number of viable leukocytes latently infected with CMV. The prevalence of CMV antibody in the donor population, the volume and the white cell contamination of the blood component transfused and the age of donor units would, therefore, influence risk. Donors who have recently experienced primary CMV infection or reactivation infection may have a larger number of latently infected leukocytes in their peripheral blood or reactivate CMV more easily.

The second factor postulated to be involved in the transmission of CMV is a cellular change such as differentiation or activation of the cell harboring latent virus. This event does not require T-cell replication as CMV has been transmitted by blood components irradiated to prevent clinical graft-vs-host disease.[24,25,50,51] The exact requirements for and mechanism involved in CMV reactivation from a latent state remain unknown. Cellular differentiation may be important. Nonpermissive embryonal carcinoma cells[52] and a human monocytic cell line[53] have become permissive for CMV when induced to differentiate. Cheung and Lang[54] suggested that allogeneic reactions associated with blood transfusion were important in the reactivation of CMV in a murine model of transfusion-acquired CMV infection. Similarly, other investigators found that cocultivation of latently infected murine mononuclear cells with allogeneic cells was required for the release of infectious CMV.[55] However, another study was unable to confirm these findings.[56]

Cultured human T lymphocytes can produce small amounts of CMV after in vitro infection following stimulation in allogeneic but not autologous mixed lymphocyte culture.[57] Recently, Chou found that in seropositive recipients of seropositive donor organs, CMV was preferentially reactivated from the donor organ compared to reactivation of endogenous CMV in the recipient.[58] Again, this suggests that local "allogeneic" factors may be more important than global immunosuppression in reactivating latent virus. Studies in a rat model of renal transplantation and CMV infection support this hypothesis.[59] A subclinical graft-vs-host reaction in donor lymphocytes appears to be a common event after blood transfusion.[60] The requirement for large numbers of transfusions and immunodeficiency in the recipient would increase the probability of this reaction, which may be a necessary initial step for CMV reactivation.

The third requirement for the transmission of CMV infection by transfusion may be survival of infected donor cells for a sufficient period of time to allow production of infectious CMV. In the setting of organ transplantation, pretransplant blood transfusions are known to promote allograft survival.[41] In the patient repetitively transfused, similar immune mechanisms may be allowing longer survival of transfused cells and reactivation and production of infectious CMV. Chou found possible evidence for this effect in the high incidence of CMV infection observed in patients receiving two transfusions of donor-specific leukocytes compared to patients receiving a similar number of leukocytes from random donors.[50] Braun and Reiser observed that CMV could be consistently isolated from T cells infected in vitro and stimulated by mitogens or allogeneic mixed lymphocyte culture if their survival time was prolonged by culture in IL-2.[57]

Donor lymphocytes have been demonstrated to persist for long periods of time in neonates, particularly in those infants who had received transfusions in utero.[61] Whether similar longevity of donor cells occurs in patients receiving exogenous immunosuppression and those who are functionally immunocompromised by the stress of burns, surgery or major trauma is not known. A high incidence of symptomatic transfusion-acquired CMV infection has been observed in the highly transfused splenectomized patient.[62,63] Whether splenectomy prolongs donor leukocyte survival is uncertain.

What Can We Learn From the Incidence of Transfusion-Acquired CMV Infection in Other Patient Populations?

In order to evaluate the studies of transfusion-acquired CMV infection in neonates, the incidence of infection documented in these studies should be compared to that observed in other patient populations.

The Immunocompetent Patient

Since the mid 1960's many studies have been undertaken to determine the incidence of transfusion-acquired CMV infection in immunocompetent populations. The results of these studies have recently been extensively reviewed.[5-7] Many of these early studies were carried out in patients undergoing cardiovascular surgery[7] and were complicated by the inclusion of allograft recipients[41] and patients who were sero-positive prior to transfusion.[7] The incidence of CMV infection documented in these studies was high with 16-67% of patients developing infection.[7] However, a change appears to have occurred in the 1970's and 1980's in the epidemiology of transfusion-acquired CMV infection.

Two recent studies examined the incidence of transfusion-acquired CMV infection in a large number of seronegative transfusion recipients and found it to be extremely low.[48,49] Wilhelm et al[48] demonstrated CMV infection in only 7 (1.2%) of 595 patients and we[49] documented CMV infection in only 6 (0.9%) of 637 transfusion recipients. The lower seroprevalence in the donor population, the older age of many of the red cell components used in these studies and the increased use of plasma may all have contributed to the lower incidence observed. The highly transfused patient is at highest risk. Despite the fact that some morbidity has been associated with primary CMV infection in immunocompetent populations, illness is generally mild and self-limited.[7]

Allograft Recipients

Cytomegalovirus remains the most common infectious complication occurring after allogeneic/autologous bone marrow[24] and solid organ transplantation.[64-77] It is difficult to determine the true incidence of transfusion-acquired CMV infection in these patients because endogenous CMV is often reactivated in the seropositive transplant recipient and CMV is transmitted by bone marrow[25] and solid organs[58] from seropositive donors. More detailed information is provided in the preceding chapter.

From incidence of transfusion-acquired CMV infection in other populations it appears that the risk is low in the immunocompetent adult. The risk also appears to be surprisingly low in some groups of heavily transfused immunosuppressed solid organ transplant recipients.

How Can We Explain the Geographic Variability in Risk of Transfusion-Acquired CMV Infections in Neonatal Populations?

Donor Factors

The disparate results observed cannot be attributed to differences in donor CMV IgG antibody prevalence (Table 6-1). Sero-prevalence rates in centers that have reported a high incidence of infection are very similar to those reporting a low incidence. Lamberson[11] and Demmler[37] have suggested that transfusion-acquired CMV infection in the neonate is linked to the receipt of blood from a CMV IgM-positive donor. Although significant differences in the seroprevalence of CMV-specific IgM have been described,[11,36,37] this is far more likely due to differences in the sensitivity of the assays used than due to true differences in seroprevalence. Significant differences in CMV IgM sero-prevalence are unlikely to occur in centers that have comparable CMV IgG seroprevalence, although this requires further study.

Red cells used for neonatal transfusions are usually fresher than those used in adult patients. This may result in a higher risk of transfusion-acquired CMV infection in neonates. However, comparably aged blood (<6 days old) was used in all the prospective neonatal studies.[8-13] The age of transfused blood is, therefore, unlikely to account for the differences observed. Details regarding the use of plasma and platelet products are not clearly documented in many of the published studies.[8-11,13] It is possible that the use of plasma in some nurseries may be reducing the risk of transfusion-acquired CMV infection through the passive administration of CMV antibody, as has been suggested by Beneke et al in adult patients.[36] Although the relative risk of platelet units versus red cell units is unknown, differences in policies regarding the use of platelets in neonatal nurseries may be altering risk. Although often not stated, it is assumed that neonates in the studies did not receive granulocyte transfusions, which would significantly increase the risk of transfusion-acquired CMV infection. Detailed comparison of blood component use in centers with high and low incidences of infection would eliminate some of these possibilities.

In two studies[9,13] in which a high incidence of transfusion-acquired CMV infection was observed, infected neonates were found to have been exposed to a larger number of donors than uninfected neonates. However, the mean number of donor exposures experienced by the neonates in the study of Preiksaitis et al,[12] who observed a low incidence of infection, was not significantly different from that reported in two centers that observed a high incidence of infection. Similarly, neither Lamberson[11] nor Tegtmeier[21] found any significant difference in the number of donor exposures between infected and uninfected infants in their studies. Adler et al[19] also found that infected neonates were exposed to a disproportionately larger number of seropositive blood donors and Yeager et al[8] suggested that the volume of blood received was important. However, in four low-birth-weight infants in two studies[11,13] CMV infection was acquired after a single exposure to a relatively small volume of blood from a single seropositive donor. Exposure to a large volume of seropositive blood and multiple seropositive donors does not appear to be necessary for the transmission of CMV infection to neonates.

Recipient Factors

Low birth weight and immaturity in the sick premature neonate are often closely linked to a large number of donor exposures. Identifying donor exposures as a risk factor may simply be identifying the host risk factor of gestational age and low birth weight. It is striking that in the three studies that have studied infants of all birth weights and reported a high incidence of transfusion-acquired CMV infection, the infection is seen almost exclusively in the very low-birth-weight infant (<1200-1500 g).[8,9,13] It is not clear from the data analysis whether these infants are at significantly higher risk of acquiring infection per seropositive donor exposure or unit volume of seropositive blood received when compared to infants of higher birth weight. If this is the case, it would point to host factors as the important determinants of risk.

Very low-birth-weight infants (<1250 g) usually have a gestational age of less than 29 weeks. These infants are immunologically immature both with respect to humoral[78] and cell-mediated immune responses.[79] Circulating donor lymphocytes persisted for very short periods of time and were never seen beyond 6-8 weeks after transfusion in term and near-term neonates receiving exchange transfusions of banked blood but were observed for over 2 years in some infants who had received fetal-maternal transfusions.[61] Survival of the leukocyte in the recipient may be necessary for the reactivation and replication of CMV in transfusion recipients. The very low-birth-weight infant may closely resemble a fetally transfused infant even though random donor cells may not survive as long as more antigenically similar maternal cells. Prolonged survival of donor cells in these infants may significantly increase their risk of acquiring CMV infection.

Transfusion-acquired graft-vs-host disease has been described in the exchange-transfused and premature infant.[79] This diagnosis may be difficult to make in the sick premature infant. Allogeneic reactions by donor lymphocytes may be more common in these immunologically immature infants even in the absence of fatal graft-vs-host disease and may be important for the reactivation of latent CMV.

In most studies of transfusion-acquired CMV infection in neonates, analysis of risk is based on the total donor exposure prior to infection.[8-13] A more important factor may be exposure to seropositive blood during a critical period of maximum immaturity in the neonate. Differences in indications for transfusions between nurseries in these infants early in their course may be significantly altering risk.

The method of blood distribution in nurseries may also influence leukocyte survival after blood transfusion in the recipient. When a syringe and aliquot technique is used in the nursery, the infant may be repetitively exposed to blood from the same donor. If the donor is seropositive, not only would the risk of exposure to a cell latently infected with CMV be increased, the survival of white cells from second or subsequent transfusions from that donor may be prolonged as has been described in the use of blood transfusions for the promotion of allograft survival. Repetitive transfusions from random donors may also have this effect. Immunotolerance induced by repetitive transfusions may be a more relevant factor in the immunologically more mature full term neonate. Two such infants who acquired CMV from blood transfusion have been described by Lamberson et al.[11]

Which Neonates Should Receive CMV-"Safe" Blood Components?

The variability in the incidence and morbidity of transfusion-acquired CMV infection makes firm recommendations regarding the need for CMV-seronegative or leukocyte-depleted blood components for neonates difficult. In centers where a high incidence of transfusion-acquired CMV infection has been identified, it would appear to be reasonable to assume that the provision of CMV-"safe" blood to very low-birth-weight (<1500 g) infants born to seronegative mothers would have a significant impact on the incidence of transfusion-acquired CMV infection and its associated morbidity and mortality. Although transfusion-acquired CMV infection has been reported to have occurred in a few higher birth weight neonates,[8,11] no symptoms could be attributed to the infection. These infants appear to more closely resemble the full-term infant who acquires CMV infection from a maternal source. Although the long-term sequelae of CMV infection in these infants remain unknown, and these infants are a potential source of infection to their seronegative mothers, there are insufficient data to support the policy of providing CMV-"safe" blood to seronegative infants with birth weights greater than 1500 g.

In many centers, CMV-seronegative blood is given to all neonates or low-birth-weight neonates without regard to their serologic status. Infants born to seropositive mothers are at risk of acquiring CMV infection from maternal genital secretions and breast milk as well as blood transfusion.[18] Yeager et al[8] found no difference in the incidence of CMV infection in neonates receiving CMV-seronegative blood and those receiving unscreened blood. These infants appear to be protected by maternally derived passive antibody and most infants, even those with low birth weights, have remained asymptomatic when infected.[8,12] In two studies of transfused infants given random blood components two of seven (both with birth weights <1250 g)[22] and two of nine infants (birth weights not reported)[11] born to seropositive mothers developed symptoms concomitant with the onset of CMV infection. It is not known whether these infections were acquired from blood transfusion.

The low-birth-weight infant of low gestational age often has very little maternal antibody, which can be depleted rapidly by venipuncture and the delutional effects of blood transfusion. Yeager et al[80] suggested that the loss of maternal CMV antibody, which may be hastened by the delutional effect of administration of seronegative blood to low-birth-weight seropositive infants, may result in earlier virus shedding and a subsequent increased risk of symptomatic CMV infection as the result of exposure to infected maternal genital secretions or breast milk. Others, however, have found no association between antibody levels and symptomatic CMV infection in full-term infants.[81] Present evidence does not support the policy of providing CMV-"safe" blood components to infants born to seropositive mothers. Further studies are required in the low-birth-weight seropositive infant in order to determine the morbidity in this subgroup of infants and validate Yeager's observations that the use of seronegative blood components may be increasing their risk of morbidity.

In centers that have documented a low incidence of transfusion-acquired CMV infection in neonates and those that have not documented any incidence, recommendations for the use of CMV-seronegative blood components are more controversial and remain uncertain. It can be argued that the prevention of a single neonatal death, even if this is a relatively infrequent event, warrants the use of CMV-seronegative blood components in low-birth-weight seronegative infants.

Although full-term neonates who acquire CMV infection after birth are usually asymptomatic and have no long-term consequences as a result of the infection, it is not known whether the low-birth-weight premature neonate who has a self-limited syndrome associated with transfusion-acquired CMV infection will develop the late neurological sequelae and hearing loss that have been documented in patients with congenital CMV infection.[18] A recent study has suggested that pneumonitis occurring in the first 3 months of life, including CMV pneumonitis, may contribute to the development of chronic obstructive airways disease in later life.[82] Sawyer et al[83] also found a possible association between CMV infection and the development of bronchopulmonary dysplasia in premature infants.

CMV infection in neonates has also been associated with prolonged hospitalization. CMV is known to be immunosuppressive.[84] Adler et al[9] have suggested that children with transfusion-acquired CMV infection may be at higher risk of superinfection with other pathogens compared to uninfected infants. This increased risk of superinfection has been observed in allograft recipients.[84] Seronegative mothers of infants with transfusion-acquired CMV infection are also at high risk of acquiring CMV infection from their infected infants with significant consequences if pregnant.[11,85] Despite these concerns, it is difficult to justify the use of seronegative blood in nurseries where transfusion-acquired CMV infection is an extremely rare event.

Indications for the use of granulocyte transfusions in the neonate are infrequent and controversial.[86] Although the incidence of transfusion-acquired CMV infection associated with granulocyte transfusions in the neonate is unknown, extrapolation of data from bone marrow transplant recipients[24,25] suggests that the risk of transmission of CMV infection is high and passive antibody is less likely to protect against CMV-associated morbidity in this setting.[87] It would, therefore, appear prudent that CMV-seronegative granulocyte transfusions be provided for both seronegative and seropositive sick premature neonates.

Extracorporeal membrane oxygenation (ECMO) has recently been introduced into neonatal nurseries for treatment of some term or near-term infants. These infants sometimes have significant transfusion requirements. In our center, in which a low incidence of transfusion-acquired CMV infection has been found in neonates, a case of presumptive transfusion-acquired CMV infection resulting in the death of an infant who had received ECMO therapy has been documented (Feiner N, personal communication). This infant was born to a seronegative mother at 36 weeks' gestation, weighing 2910 g. Evidence of disseminated CMV infection was present on postmortem examination. This child had received a total 47 red cell, 34 platelet, 76 plasma and 31 cryoprecipitate transfusions during his hospital course prior to death. The birth weight of this child would not have placed him in a high risk category for symptomatic transfusion-acquired CMV infection. Further data are required regarding the risk of transfusion-acquired CMV infection and its morbidity in infants treated with ECMO. This group of patients may be a subset that would benefit from the use of seronegative or leukocyte-depleted blood components.

The proven indications for the use of CMV-"safe" blood components must be balanced against the logistics of providing these components to subgroups of infants in the nursery. Priorities for the distribution of these components are outlined in Table 6-3.

Alternatives to the Use of Seronegative Cellular Blood Components

The use of serologic screening of blood donors for CMV-specific IgG and the elimination of cellular blood components from these donors for use in high risk populations have been very effective in significantly reducing and even eliminating the risk of transfusion-acquired CMV infection.[8,88] Several commercially available serologic techniques are both practical and sensitive enough for large-scale screening in blood banks. These techniques include latex agglutination, indirect hemagglutination (IHA), indirect immunofluorescence, solid-phase fluorescence immunoassays and enzyme-linked immunoassay (EIA).[7]

Table 6-3. Indications for the Use of CMV-Seronegative Cellular Blood Components

Category A (populations in whom the use of CMV-seronegative cellular blood components have been proven to reduce the incidence and morbidity of CMV infection using controlled trials)

- low-birth-weight infants born to seronegative mothers in centers that have documented a high incidence of transfusion-acquired infection in neonates.

Category B (populations at high risk of significant morbidity as the result of transfusion-acquired CMV infection, but the incidence of transfusion-acquired CMV infection in these populations has not been clearly documented and the benefit of using CMV-seronegative cellular blood components has not been proven)

- low-birth-weight infants born to seronegative or seropositive mothers requiring granulocyte transfusions

- neonates receiving ECMO (extracorporeal membrane oxygenation)

Category C (populations in which the incidence and/or morbidity of transfusion-acquired CMV infection is low or poorly documented)

- low-birth-weight infants born to seronegative mothers in centers that have documented a low incidence of transfusion-acquired infection in neonates

- low-birth-weight infants born to seropositive mothers in centers that have documented a high incidence of transfusion-acquired infection in neonates

- infants with birth weights >1500 g born to seronegative mothers

Category D (populations in which the incidence and morbidity associated with transfusion-acquired CMV infection is low, the use of CMV-seronegative cellular blood components is probably not indicated)

- infants with birth weights >1500 g born to seropositive mothers

Because there is no "gold standard" serological test for CMV seropositivity, no single test will be 100% sensitive. A small number of seropositive components will remain undetected and may transmit CMV infection. This risk appears to be low and it has been estimated that by the latex agglutination test for example, only 1.1% of sera are falsely negative.[88] Mononuclear cells from some blood donors were found to be repetitively positive for CMV DNA despite negative CMV serology using a PCR assay.[34] However, further studies to determine the sensitivity and specificity of PCR assays are required before it can be considered as an alternative to serological testing. Similarly, the use of assays for CMV-specific IgM to select out a subgroup of "infectious" seropositive blood donors cannot be recommended at the present time.

In centers where the donor seroprevalence is high or populations requiring seronegative cellular blood components are large, maintenance of adequate supplies of seronegative blood components may be extremely difficult. There is increasing evidence that the effective removal of leukocytes from cellular blood components will eliminate the risk of transfusion-acquired CMV infection. What is unknown is how effective leukocyte removal must be in order to render a product CMV-"safe." Lang et al[89] first tested this hypothesis in 1977 by comparing the incidence of transfusion-acquired CMV infection in patients receiving fresh whole blood to those receiving leukocyte-poor blood (60% leukocyte removal by an inverted spin procedure). The incidence of CMV infection was reduced but not eliminated. Demmler et al[37] found that saline washing of red cells did not prevent CMV infection in neonates, although three of the six infants she studied had also received seropositive standard platelet transfusions.

Other investigators found that infants at their center receiving saline-washed red cells had a very low incidence of CMV infection.[90] However, the incidence of CMV infection at that center in infants receiving standard blood components was not documented. The efficacy of saline washing of red cells to reduce the risk of CMV infection remains uncertain. The use of frozen deglycerolized red cells has been shown to have significantly reduced the risk of CMV infection in neonates[22,40,91] and dialysis patients[92] when compared to historical controls at the same and other centers. The use of leukocyte filters has been demonstrated to eliminate the risk of transfusion-acquired CMV infection in neonates,[13] bone marrow transplant recipients[93] and patients with leukemia,[94] although the latter two studies were uncontrolled. Preliminary evidence suggests that differential centrifugation of platelet units may also render them CMV-"safe."[76,95]

There are an increasing number of methods that can be used to provide CMV-"safe" blood to patients. It is possible to eliminate the problem of transfusion-acquired infection in all patients, but the expense of doing so would be prohibitive. It is important to establish which subgroups of patients are most likely to benefit from these programs. The complexity of transfusion-acquired CMV infection is illustrated by this discussion of the problem in neonates. A better understanding of the pathogenesis of transfusion-acquired CMV infection may allow a better explanation of these differences, more accurately define patient populations at risk and provide clear guidelines that can be universally applied regarding who should receive CMV-"safe" blood.

Acknowledgments

I would like to thank Dr. J. Hanon and Dr. J. Culver-James for providing the transfusion medicine perspective in useful discussions.

References

1. Purcell RP. Hepatitis B: A scientific success story (almost). In: Dodd RY, Barker LF, eds. Infection, immunity and blood transfusion. New York: Alan R. Liss, Inc, 1985:11-43.
2. Alter HJ, Purcell RH, Shih JW, et al. Detection of antibody to hepatitis C virus in prospectively followed transfusion recipients with acute and chronic non-A,non-B hepatitis. N Engl J Med 1989;321:1494-500.
3. Feorino PM, Jaffe HW, Palmer E, et al. Transfusion-associated acquired immunodeficiency syndrome: Evidence for persistent infection in blood donors. N Engl J Med 1985;312:1293-6.
4. Menitove JE. The decreasing risk of transfusion-associated AIDS. N Engl J Med 1989;321:966-8.
5. Adler SP. Transfusion-associated cytomegalovirus infections. Rev Infect Dis 1983;5:977-93.
6. Tegtmeier GE. Cytomegalovirus and blood transfusion. In: Dodd RY, Barker LF, eds. Infection, immunity and blood transfusion. New York: Alan R. Liss, Inc, 1985:175-99.
7. Tegtmeier GE. Posttransfusion cytomegalovirus infections. Arch Pathol Lab Med 1989;13:236-45.
8. Yeager AS, Grumet FC, Hafleigh EB, et al. Prevention of transfusion-acquired cytomegalovirus infections in newborn infants. J Pediatr 1981;98:281-7.
9. Adler SP, Chandrika T, Lawrence L, Baggett J. Cytomegalovirus infections in neonates acquired by blood transfusions. Pediatr Infect Dis J 1983;2:114-18.

10. Smith D Jr, Wright P, Krueger L, et al. Posttransfusion cytomegalovirus infection in neonates weighing less than 1250 grams (abstract). Transfusion 1983;23:420.
11. Lamberson HV, McMillan JA, Weiner LB, et al. Prevention of transfusion associated cytomegalovirus (CMV) infection in neonates by screening blood donors for IgM to CMV. J Infect Dis 1988;157:820-3.
12. Preiksaitis JK, Brown L, McKenzie M. Transfusion-acquired cytomegalovirus infection in neonates: A prospective study. Transfusion 1988;28:205-9.
13. Gilbert GL, Hayes K, Hudson IL, James J. Prevention of transfusion-acquired cytomegalovirus infection in infants by blood filtration to remove leucocytes. Lancet 1989;2: 1228-31.
14. Kumar A, Nankervis GA, Cooper AR, et al. Acquisition of cytomegalovirus infection in infants following exchange transfusion: A prospective study. Transfusion 1980;20: 327-31.
15. Benson JWT, Bodden SJ, Tobin JO. Cytomegalovirus and blood transfusion in neonates. Arch Dis Child 1979:54: 538-41.
16. Yeager AS. Transfusion-acquired cytomegalovirus infection in newborn infants. Am J Dis Child 1974;128:478-83.
17. Spector SA, Schmidt K, Ticknor W, Grossman M. Cytomegaloviruria in older infants in intensive care nurseries. J Pediatr 1979;95:444-6.
18. Stagno S, Pass RF, Dworsky ME, Alford CA. Congenital and perinatal cytomegaloviral infections. Semin Perinatol 1983;7:31-42.
19. Ballard RA, Drew WL, Hufnagle KG, Riedel PA. Acquired cytomegalovirus infection in preterm infants. Am J Dis Child 1979;133:482-5.
20. Pass MA, Johnson JD, Schulman IA, et al. Evaluation of a walking donor blood transfusion program in an intensive care nursery. J Pediatr 1976;89:646-51.
21. Tegtmeier GE. Transfusion-acquired CMV infection in premature infants. Transfusion 1989;29:279.
22. Adler SP, Lawrence LT, Baggett J, et al. Prevention of transfusion-associated cytomegalovirus infections in very low birth weight infants using frozen blood and donors seronegative for cytomegalovirus. Transfusion 1984;24: 333-5.
23. Tolpin MD, Stewart JA, Warren D, et al. Transfusion transmission of cytomegalovirus confirmed by restriction endonuclease analysis. J Pediatr 1985;107:953-6.

24. Winston DJ, Ho WG, Howell CL, et al. Cytomegalovirus infections associated with leukocyte transfusions. Ann Intern Med 1980;93:671-5.

25. Meyers JD, Flournoy N, Thomas ED. Risk factors for cytomegalovirus infection after human marrow transplantation. J Infect Dis 1986;3:478-88.

26. Rinaldo CV, Black PH, Hirsch MS. Interaction of cytomegalovirus with leukocytes from patients with mononucleosis due to cytomegalovirus. J Infect Dis 1977;136: 667-78.

27. Turtinen LR, Saltzman M, Jordan M, Haase A. Interactions of human cytomegalovirus with leukocytes in vivo: Analysis by in situ hybridization. Microb Pathog 1987;3: 287-97.

28. Dankner WM, McCutchan A, Richman DD, et al. Localization of human cytomegalovirus in peripheral blood leukocytes by in situ hybridization. J Infect Dis 1990;161: 31-6.

29. Diosi P, Moldovan E, Tomescu N. Latent cytomegalovirus infection in blood donors. Br Med J 1969;4:660-2.

30. Einhorn L, Ost A. Cytomegalovirus infection of human blood cells. J Infect Dis 1984;149:207-14.

31. Rice GPA, Schrier RD, Oldstone MBA. Cytomegalovirus infects human lymphocytes and monocytes: Virus expression is restricted to immediate-early gene products. Proc Natl Acad Sci USA 1984;81:6134-8.

32. Rinaldo CR, Richter BS, Black PH, et al. Replication of herpes simplex virus and cytomegalovirus in human leukocytes. J Immunol 1978;120:130-6.

33. Schrier RD, Nelson JA, Oldstone MBA. Detection of human cytomegalovirus in peripheral blood lymphocytes in a natural infection. Science 1985;230:1048-51.

34. Stanier P, Taylor DL, Kitchen AD, et al. Persistence of cytomegalovirus in mononuclear cells in peripheral blood from blood donors. Br Med J 1989;299:897-8.

35. Toorkey CB, Carrigan DR. Immunohistochemical detection of immediate early antigen of human cytomegalovirus in normal tissues. J Infect Dis 1989;160:741-51.

36. Beneke JS, Tegtmeier GE, Alter HJ, et al. Relation of titers of antibodies to CMV in blood donors to the transmission of cytomegalovirus infection. J Infect Dis 1984;150:883-8.

37. Demmler GJ, Brady MT, Bijou H, et al. Posttransfusion cytomegalovirus infections in neonates: Role of saline-washed red cells. J Pediatr 1986;108:762-65.

38. McVoy MA, Adler SP. Immunologic evidence for frequent age-related cytomegalovirus reactivation in seropositive

immunocompetent individuals. J Infect Dis 1989;160:1-10.

39. D'Addosio AM, Fagiolo E. T lymphocyte content in blood components. Haematologica 1986;71:379-81.

40. Brady MT, Milam JT, Anderson DC, et al. Use of deglycerolized red cells to prevent posttransfusion infection with cytomegalovirus in neonates. J Infect Dis 1984; 150:334-9.

41. Prince HE, Arens L. Effect of storage on lymphocyte surface markers in whole blood units. Transplantation 1986; 41:235-8.

42. Dzik WH, Neckers L. Lymphocyte subpopulations altered during blood storage. N Engl J Med 1983;309:435-6.

43. Paloheimo JA, von Essen R, Klemola E, et al. Subclinical cytomegalovirus infections and cytomegalovirus mononucleosis after open heart surgery. Am J Cardiol 1968;22:624-30.

44. Stevens DP, Barker LF, Ketcham AS, Meyer HM Jr. Asymptomatic cytomegalovirus infection following blood transfusion in tumor surgery. JAMA 1970;211:1341-4.

45. Prince AM, Szmuness W, Millian SJ, David DS. A serologic study of cytomegalovirus infections associated with blood transfusions. N Engl J Med 1971;284:1125-31.

46. Medical Research Council (MRC) Working Party on Post-Transfusion Hepatitis. Report to the MRC Blood Transfusion Research Committee. Post-transfusion hepatitis in a London hospital: Results of a two-year prospective study. J Hyg 1974;75:173-88.

47. Monif GRG, Daicoff GI, Flory LF. Blood as a potential vehicle for the cytomegaloviruses. Am J Obstet Gynecol 1976;126:445-8.

48. Wilhelm JA, Matter L, Schopfer K. The risk of transmitting cytomegalovirus to patients receiving blood transfusion. J Infect Dis 1986;154:169-71.

49. Preiksaitis JK, Brown L, McKenzie M. The risk of cytomegalovirus infection in seronegative transfusion recipients not receiving exogenous immunosuppression. J Infect Dis 1988;157:523-9.

50. Chou S, Kim DY, Norman DJ. Transmission of cytomeg-alovirus by pretransplant leukocyte transfusions in renal transplant candidates. J Infect Dis 1987;155:565-7.

51. Bowden RA, Sayers M, Flournoy N, et al. Cytomegalovirus immune globulin and seronegative blood products to prevent primary cytomegalovirus infection after marrow transplantation. N Engl J Med 1986;314:1006-10.

52. Gonczol E, Andrews PW, Plotkin SA. Cytomegalovirus replicates in differentiated but not in undifferentiated human embryonal carcinoma cells. Science 1984;224:159-61.

53. Weinshenker BG, Wilton S, Rice GP. Phorbol ester-induced differentiation permits productive human cytomegalovirus infection in a monocytic cell line. J Immunol 1988;140: 1625-31.

54. Cheung KS, Lang DJ. Transmission and activation of cytomegalovirus with blood transfusion: A mouse model. J Infect Dis 1977;135:841-5.

55. Olding LB, Jensen FC, Oldstone MBA. Pathogenesis of cytomegalovirus infection. I. Activation of virus from bone marrow-derived lymphocytes by in vitro allogenic reaction. J Exp Med 1975;141:561-720.

56. Jordan MC, Mar VL. Spontaneous activation of latent cytomegalovirus from murine speen explants: Role of lymphocytes and macrophages in release and replication of virus. J Clin Invest 1982;70:762-8.

57. Braun RW, Reiser HC. Replication of human cytomegalovirus in peripheral blood T cells. J Virol 1986; 60:29-36.

58. Chou S. Neutralizing antibody responses to reinfecting strains of cytomegalovirus in transplant recipients. J Infect Dis 1989;160:16-21.

59. Bruning JH, Bruggeman CA, Van Boven CPA, et al. Reactivation of latent rat cytomegalovirus by a combination of immunosuppression and administration of allogeneic immunocompetent cells. Transplantation 1989;47:917-18.

60. Schecter GP, Whang-Peng J, McFarland W. Circulation of donor lymphocytes after blood transfusion in man. Blood 1977;49:651-6.

61. Hutchinson DL, Turner JH, Schlesinger ER. Persistence of donor cells in neonates after fetal and exchange transfusion. Am J Obstet Gynecol 1971;109:281-4.

62. Baumgartner JD, Glauser MP, Burgo-Black AL, et al. Severe cytomegalovirus infection in multiply transfused, splenectomized, trauma patients. Lancet 1982;2:63-6.

63. Drew WL, Miner RC. Transfusion-related cytomegalovirus infection following noncardiac surgery. JAMA 1982;247: 2389-91.

64. Rubin RH, Tolkoff-Rubin NE, Older R, et al. Multicenter seroepidemiologic study of the impact of cytomegalovirus infection on renal transplantation. Transplantation 1985; 40:243-9.

65. Marker SC, Howard RJ, Simmons RL, et al. Cytomegalovirus infection: A quantitative prospective study of three

hundred twenty consecutive renal transplants. Surgery 1981;89:660-71.

66. Boyce NW, Hayes K, Gee D, et al. Cytomegalovirus infection complicating renal transplantation and its relationship to acute transplant glomerulopathy. Transplantation 1988;45:706-9.

67. Harris KR, Saeed AA, Digard NJ, et al. Cytomegalovirus titers in kidney transplant donor and recipient: Influence of cyclosporine A. Transplant Proc 1984;16:31-3.

68. Chou S, Norman DJ. The influence of donor factors other than serologic status on transmission of cytomegalovirus to transplant recipients. Transplantation 1988;46:89-93.

69. Kurtz JK, Thompson JF, Ting A, et al. The problem of cytomegalovirus infection in renal allograft recipients. J Med 1984:New Series LIII:341-9.

70. Smiley ML, Wlodaver CG, Grossman RA, et al. The role of pretransplant immunity in protection from cytomegalovirus disease following renal transplantation. Transplantation 1985;40:157-61.

71. Preiksaitis JK, Rosno S, Grumet C, Merigan TC. Infections due to herpesviruses in cardiac transplant recipients: Role of the donor heart and immunosuppressive therapy. J Infect Dis 1983;147:974-81.

72. Wreghitt TG, Hakim M, Gray JJ, et al. Cytomegalovirus infections in heart and heart and lung transplant recipients. J Clin Pathol 1988;41:660-7.

73. Singh N, Dummer JS, Kusne S, et al. Infections with cytomegalovirus and other herpesviruses in 121 liver transplant recipients: Transmission by donated organ and the effect of OKT3 antibodies. J Infect Dis 1993;158:124-31.

74. Wingard JR, Chen DYH, Burns WH, et al. Cytomegalovirus infection after autologous bone marrow transplantation with comparison to infection after allogeneic bone marrow transplantation. Blood 1993;71:1432-7.

75. Bowden RA, Sayers M, Slichter SJ, Meyers JD. Use of leukocyte-poor transfusions to prevent transfusion-associated cytomegalovirus (CMV) infection after marrow transplant (abstract). Second international herpes virus workshop, San Diego, March 1989. San Diego: University of California 1989:67.

76. Rakela J, Taswell HF, Hermans PE, et al. Incidence of cytomegalovirus infection and its relationship to donor-recipient serologic status in liver transplantation. Transplant Proc 1987;19:2399-402.

77. Gorensek MJ, Stewart RW, Keys TF, et al. A multivariate analysis of the risk of cytomegalovirus infection in heart transplant recipients. J Infect Dis 1988;157:515-22.
78. Conway SP, Dear PRF, Smith I. Immunoglobulin profile of the preterm baby. Arch Dis Child 1985;60:208-12.
79. Holland PV. Transfusion-associated graft-versus-host disease: Prevention using irradiated blood products. In: Garratty G, ed. Current concepts in transfusion therapy. Arlington, VA: American Association of Blood Banks, 1985: 295-315.
80. Yeager AS, Palumbo PE, Malachowski N, et al. Sequelae of maternally derived cytomegalovirus infections in premature infants. J Pediatr 1983;102:918-22.
81. Kumar ML, Nankervis GA, Cooper AR, Gold E. Postnatally acquired cytomegalovirus infections in infants of CMV-excreting mothers. J Pediatr 1984;104:669-73.
82. Basfield DM, Stagno S, Whitley RJ, et al. Infant pneumonitis associated with cytomegalovirus, chlamydia, pneumocystis and ureaplasma: Follow up. Pediatrics 1987;79:76-93.
83. Sawyer MH, Edward DK, Spector SA. Cytomegalovirus infection and bronchopulmonary dysplasia in premature infants. Am J Dis Child 1987;141:303-5.
84. Rand KH, Pollard RB, Merigan TC. Increased pulmonary superinfections in cardiac transplant patients undergoing primary cytomegalovirus infection. N Engl J Med 1978; 298:951-3.
85. Yeager AS. Transmission of cytomegalovirus to mothers by infected infants: Another reason to prevent transfusion-acquired infections. Pediatr Infect Dis 1983;2:295-7.
86. Strauss RG. Current issues in neonatal transfusions. Vox Sang 1986;51:1-9.
87. Meyers JD, Leszczynski J, Zaia JA, et al. Prevention of cytomegalovirus infection by cytomegalovirus immune globulin after marrow transplantation. Ann Intern Med 1983;98:442-6.
88. Bowden RA, Sayers M, Gleaves CA, et al. Cytomegalovirus-seronegative blood components for the prevention of primary cytomegalovirus infection after marrow transplantation. Considerations for blood banks. Transfusion 1987; 27:478-81.
89. Lang, DJ, Ebert PA, Rodgers BM, et al. Reductions of post-perfusion cytomegalovirus infections following the use of leucocyte-depleted blood. Transfusion 1977;17: 391-5.

90. Luban NLC, Williams AE, McDonald M, et al. Low inci-
    dence of cytomegalovirus infection in neonates transfused
    with washed red blood cells. Am J Dis Child 1987; 141:
    416-19.
91. Taylor BJ, Jacobs RF, Baker RL, et al. Frozen degly-
    cerolized blood prevents transfusion-acquired cytomegalo-
    virus infections in neonates. Pediatr Infect Dis 1986;5:
    188-91.
92. Tolkoff-Rubin NE, Rubin RH, Keller EE, et al. Cytomega-
    lovirus infection in dialysis patients and personnel. Ann
    Intern Med 1978;89:625-8.
93. Verdonck LF, de Graan-Hentzen AW, Dekker AW, et al.
    Cytomegalovirus seronegative platelets and leukocyte-
    poor red blood cells from random donors can prevent
    primary cytomegalovirus infection after bone marrow
    transplantation. Bone Marrow Transplantation 1987;2:
    73-8.
94. de Graan-Hentzen YCE, Gratama JW, Mudde GC, et al.
    Prevention of primary cytomegalovirus (CMV) infection
    during induction treatment of acute leukaemia using at
    random leucocyte poor blood products (abstract). Br J
    Haematol 1987;66:421.
95. Murphy MF, Grint PCA, Hardiman AE, et al. Use of leuco-
    cyte-poor components to prevent primary cytomegalovirus
    (CMV) infection in patients with acute leukaemia. Br J
    Haematol 1988;70:253-4.

In Kurtz SR, Baldwin ML and Sirchia G, eds.
Controversies in Transfusion Medicine:
Immune Complications and Cytomegalovirus Transmission
Arlington, VA: American Association
of Blood Banks, 1990

7

Cytomegalovirus-Seronegative Blood Support for Perinatal Patients—PRO

Nancy L. Dock, PhD

THIS TEXTBOOK CENTERS ON two types of complications—those that are immune-mediated and those that are complicated by cytomegalovirus (CMV) infection. The subjects are not as unrelated as they may appear at first glance. Infectious complications of blood transfusion from CMV may have no effect on an individual with intact immunity, whereas these complications can produce life-threatening disease in a recipient who is immunocompromised. CMV plays a role in regulating the human host's immune response and may infect the immune cells as well. Immune recognition of allogeneic antigens in transfused blood may influence the activation of CMV in that blood component or in the recipient. As the unknown mechanisms that control both immune-mediated responses to transfusion and to transfusion-transmitted CMV infection become understood, we may discover that these processes have molecular regulatory pathways in common, which might help to explain some of these interactions.[1,2]

Characteristics of CMV

To address the role CMV plays in transfusion complications, it is necessary to review the prevalence, strong cell association and peculiarities of CMV transfusion transmission.

Nancy L. Dock, PhD, Scientific Director, Research and Development, American Red Cross Blood Services, Syracuse, New York

Prevalence

First, CMV has very high prevalence in the human population. Results of seroprevalence studies performed all over the world estimate that from about 40% to nearly 100% of humans are infected. This nearly ubiquitous distribution makes it impossible to manage CMV in the blood supply in the same manner as infectious agents that occur in extremely low prevalence. For example, all the blood from donors testing positive for human immunodeficiency virus (HIV) and hepatitis B virus (HBV) can be removed from the available transfusion pool without affecting supply, whereas discarding CMV-positive blood could cut the present blood supply by at least half. Fortunately, discarding CMV-positive blood is not necessary because transfusion of CMV-positive blood usually does not mean CMV infection for the recipient, nor does it result in posttransfusion disease in most transfusion recipients who become infected. Instead, only the most severely immunocompromised patients succumb to severe CMV disease following transfusion-associated CMV infection (TA-CMV). Therefore, most patients receive blood for which the CMV status is not known, while small numbers of selected patients receive blood components that are CMV-negative.

Virus-Cell Association

Another characteristic of. CMV, important for its impact on transfusion issues, is its very strong cell association. In tissue culture, conditions can be manipulated such that cell-free virus is produced abundantly, but in vivo, CMV is highly associated with leukocytes. CMV can be easily cultured from peripheral blood leukocyte preparations from symptomatic, CMV-infected individuals and can be detected in these same specimens using antibodies directed at specific CMV antigens. Although CMV rarely has been cultured from or detected in peripheral blood leukocytes from asymptomatic CMV-seropositive individuals, it is assumed that these cells harbor CMV in its latent state. Research studies aimed toward demonstrating latent CMV in peripheral blood leukocytes have been attempted, but preliminary results have not been confirmed.[3] Therefore, it is necessary to rely on experience that indicates that transfusion of noncellular blood fractions has not been shown to transmit CMV. This is indirect, but compelling, evidence for the strong association of CMV with cellular blood components. Thus, techniques such as filtration and freezing in glycerol to remove leukocytes from blood have been proposed as effective measures for preventing transfusion-associated CMV infection.

Transfusion Issues

The question for the 1990's is probably not the technical one: "Could we provide CMV-negative cellular blood components?" Rather, it is a logistical one: "Does provision of CMV-negative blood add sufficient benefit to justify the cost and potential supply limitations at this time?" In addition to balancing supply and cost constraints, the legal/medical environment, which influences transfusion medicine today, strongly drives us all to closely examine any situation where a viral infection can be transmitted by blood transfusion. Although it is desirable to seek scientific proof of transfusion-transmitted disease and clearly defined methods for transmission prevention, the legal responsibilities associated with the provision of the service may influence transfusion practices as much as scientific studies.

Neonatal Infection and Transfusion Studies

This discussion will concentrate on CMV neonatal transfusion. However, the issues raised for CMV transmission eventually must be broadened to include additional immunocompromised patients who are also at risk for TA-CMV infection, for they are more numerous than neonates and their transfusion needs will have a far greater impact on supply. The first description of posttransfusion CMV infection appearing as non-Epstein-Barr virus infectious mononucleosis was proposed by Kaariainen[4] in 1966. This was followed in 1969 by a similar description of posttransfusion CMV infectious mononucleosis-like syndrome by Foster and Jack.[5] Case descriptions of posttransfusion CMV syndrome occurring in neonates were reported in 1979 by Hanshaw,[6] Kumar,[7] Benson[8] and by Ballard,[9] who described clinical symptoms such as the "gray pallor" of neonates. The reporting of clinical symptoms was accompanied by observations that this transfusion complication occurred most commonly in premature low-birth-weight neonates and that CMV-seronegative infants were at highest risk.

In the initial 1974 report by Yeager et al,[10] populations of transfused and nontransfused neonates were studied. Her results indicated that transfused neonates acquired CMV infection significantly more often than those who were not transfused. This finding initiated more studies of the frequency of transfusion-transmitted CMV and of the clinical results of CMV infections in this population. Two studies that created the foundation for current neonatal transfusion guidelines were performed by Yeager in 1981[11] and by Adler in 1983.[12] Both of these studies showed that transfusion of CMV-seropositive blood to CMV-seronegative recipients was responsible for morbidity and mortality in the neonatal population. Yeager's group reported that of 74 seronegative infants who were transfused, 10 became infected with CMV, a rate of 13.5%. Likewise, Adler found that of 76 seronegative infants who were transfused with seropositive blood, seven, or 9.2%, became infected. Five of Yeager's 10 infected infants had symptoms of CMV infection and four of these five infants died. In Adler's study, six of seven infants had CMV-related symptoms and three of those six infants died.

Results from these two studies prompted several other studies to be performed in hospitalized neonates. At the same time, and probably because of these results, the AABB wrote standards for transfusion of neonates, which read[13]: "Where transfusion-associated cytomegalovirus (CMV) disease is a problem, components that contain formed elements should be selected or processed to reduce that risk to neonatal recipients weighing less than 1250 grams at birth, when either the neonatal recipient or the mother is CMV-antibody-negative or that information is unknown."

The initial and continuing studies of TA-CMV infections have been thoroughly discussed in excellent reviews by Adler[14,15] and Tegtmeier.[16,17] In addition, a book by Ho[18] contains a descriptive table reviewing the studies performed during the 1970's. The reader is referred to these sources. The major findings of neonate transfusion studies for the 1980's will be reviewed here.

Neonatal Transfusion Studies in the 1980's

Throughout the 1980's when prospective studies of CMV transmission were performed, serological detection assays were dramatically improved. Implementation of these assays on the donor populations supplying blood for the neonates monitored in these transfusion studies allowed for transfusion data to accumulate that supported previous findings of the variable CMV seroprevalence throughout the world. Transfusion medicine investigators were interested in establishing the incidence of CMV infection in their neonatal populations as well as the prevalence of CMV in their blood donor populations. These studies were in large part performed and published, and the findings widely debated during the 1980's. Table 7-1 represents a selection of data from each of these studies in neonates. Although each study approached the problem differently, the major study goal was to determine the incidence of transfusion-transmitted CMV infection and morbidity and

Table 7-1. Incidence of Transfusion-Transmitted CMV Infection

Author, Time and Location of Study Data	Number of Seronegative Neonates			
	Infected/ % Transfused	Symptomatic/ Infected	Deaths/ Symptomatic	Birth Weights (g)
Yeager et al (1981)[11] ('76-'78, Stanford, CA USA)	10/74 (13.5)	5/10	4/5	<1200
Adler et al (1983)[12] ('80-'82, Richmond, VA USA)	7/76 (9.2)	6/7	3/6	<1050
Rawls et al (1984)[19] ('78-'80, Hamilton, ON Canada)	1/23 (4.3)	NA*	NA	NA
Griffin et al (1988)[20] ('84-'85, Durham, NC USA)	0/72 (0)	0	0	<1250
Lamberson et al (1988)[21] ('82-'85, Syracuse, NY USA)	7/222 (3.2)	1/7	1/1	<1000
Preiksaitis et al (1988)[22] ('83-'85, Edmonton, AL Canada)	1/126 (0.8)	1/1	0/1	<1250
Smith et al (1988) (cited in ref 23) ('82-'83, Nashville, TN USA)	1/18 (5.5)	1/1	0/1	<1250
Tegtmeier et al (1988)[23] ('83-'85, Kansas City, MO USA)	2/29 (6.9)	2/2	0/2	<1500
Gilbert et al (1989)[24] ('86-'87, Melbourne, VI Australia)	9/42 (21)	5/9	1/5	<1250

*NA = Not available

mortality of the infected neonates. For this table, the number of seronegative neonates transfused with unselected blood components serves as the denominator for the number of seronegative transfused infants who acquired CMV infection. The number of infected infants who developed CMV-related symptoms, the number of resulting deaths and the birth weights of these infants are also listed on the table. Although there were not consistent criteria for "low birth weight," all infants with morbidity and mortality were <1500 g

Since data from transfusion studies are collected and presented differently, inclusion of all studies for direct comparison is not always possible. In addition to the studies presented in Table 7-1, Bhumbra et al[25] reported that 0/127 neonates with birth weights <2000 g became infected with CMV when CMV-seronegative blood donors were preselected. However, lack of specificity of a serological assay was responsible for two neonatal infections, neither of which caused CMV disease. A large study by Weston et al[26] included two seronegative neonates who probably had transfusion-associated CMV infection among the 21 of 212 transfused neonates who became infected with CMV.

Transfusion Studies Employing Preventive Measures

Some of the studies cited in Table 7-1 and additional studies evaluated the incidence of CMV infection before and after some intervention was taken to prevent CMV transmission (Table 7-2). Yeager et al[11] demonstrated complete prevention of TA-CMV infection when only seronegative blood was transfused to seronegative neonates. This finding was supported by Adler[27] and Lamberson.[21] In studies reported by Demmler et al in 1986[31] and by Luban et al in 1987,[32] both groups transfused saline-washed packed red blood cells to neonates. The study by Luban et al showed this method to be efficacious for decreasing but not preventing CMV transmission. Demmler's study reported that 11% of seronegative transfused neonates became infected in spite of washing red cells.

Transfusion of frozen deglycerolized red cells was shown several times to be efficacious for prevention of CMV transmission in neonates. Four separate studies[27-30] each performed in a different city in the United States showed similar results. Only one infant in Simon's study[30] reported an infection in a neonate who received deglycerolized red cells. In this case, the mother also seroconverted at the same time as the infant, and

Table 7-2. CMV Prevention in Seronegative Neonates

Investigator Publication Year (Reference #)	Prevention Strategy Treatment of RBC	Incidence of TA-CMV Infection Number Infected/Number Transfused	
		Control Group (%)	Prevention Group (%)
Yeager 1981 (11)	CMV seronegative	10/74 (13.5)	0/90 (0)
Adler 1984 (27)	Frozen/deglyc CMV seronegative	7/25 (28)	0/34 (0)
Brady 1984 (28)	Frozen/deglyc	NA*	0/157 (0)
Taylor 1986 (29)	Frozen/deglyc	3/9 (33.3)	0/54 (0)
Simon 1987 (30)	Frozen/deglyc	2/16 (12.5)	1/26 (3.8)
Griffin 1988 (20)	Frozen/deglyc	0/33 (0)	0/39 (0)
Demmler 1986 (31)	Saline washed	NA	6/54 (11)
Luban 1987 (32)	Saline washed	NA	1/100 (1)
Lamberson 1988 (21)	CMV IgM negative	7/222 (3.2)	1/141 (0.7)
Gilbert 1989 (24)	Filtration	9/42 (21.4)	0/30 (0)

*NA = Not available

other routes of transmission could not be entirely ruled out. Although historical controls were used for some interpretation of the results of these four studies, the efficacy of freezing and deglycerolization of red cells for infectivity to CMV is clearly supportable by these data. Whether the freezing process itself decreases the infectivity of CMV or lost viability of leukocytes is more responsible for decreasing viral transmission, this modality is an excellent option for CMV prevention.

Another type of CMV prevention attempt was made by Lamberson et al[21] who transfused only blood components that were negative for CMV IgM. The rationale of this study design was to test whether CMV IgM was a marker for the subset of seropositive donors able to transmit CMV. This study was successful in reducing the incidence of CMV infections; however, one infant transfused with antibody-positive, but IgM-negative blood did become infected. Later, in retrospective analysis of that donor's samples, IgM positivity was documented by a more sensitive assay. Implementation of IgM CMV testing in another transfusion population was reported in 1984 by Beneke et al.[33] This group did an extensive prospective evaluation of cardiac surgery patients employing CMV IgM screening of blood components, and found significant prevention of CMV transmission during the time IgM-screened blood was used. However, lack of sensitivity of available CMV IgM assays remains a problem for use in blood screening.

In a multicenter, controlled trial in hospitalized neonates, Gilbert et al[24] reported prevention of TA-CMV infections by use of filtered red cells. This study and an ongoing study by Bowden and colleagues in marrow transplant recipients[34] are the first very encouraging results for prevention of CMV transmission in these patient groups using blood components leukocyte-depleted by filtration.

Other Transfusion Studies

During the same time period that these neonatal studies were performed, several large prospective studies of transfusion-associated CMV infection were conducted in nonneonatal populations of highly transfused patients[35,36] and cardiac surgery patients[33,37] using similar techniques for preventing CMV transmission. These studies served to validate use of serological techniques that demonstrated that seronegative blood did not transmit CMV. Furthermore, these studies reported that transfusion of CMV-positive blood to adult patients caused little morbidity and no mortality. In addition, these studies have contributed significantly to determining the utility and effectiveness of several methods for providing CMV-negative blood components and have added to local donor CMV seroprevalence information.

The one adult population not thoroughly studied until recently is the population undergoing bone marrow transplantation. These individuals have extremely high morbidity and mortality following CMV infection, which is very frequently transmitted by the marrow or blood transfusions. As with the neonatal studies, prospective studies of bone marrow transplant recipients are being performed to evaluate prevention measures. The efficacy of using only seronegative blood components for these patients has been shown by MacKinnon[38] and Bowden.[39] Since the transfusion needs of this patient population can be so great, methods other than CMV-seronegative selection have been considered. Early studies using filtration techniques have shown particularly encouraging results.[40] Therefore, the two populations at highest risk for CMV infection, neonates and marrow transplant recipients, will be the testing ground for future CMV prevention technologies.

In spite of the time of performance and technique differences that all of these studies represent, there are some consistent findings that confirm a known body of knowledge about CMV transmission that can be extremely helpful for formulating transfusion policies. When CMV-seronegative blood is transfused exclusively and CMV transmission by other routes has not occurred concurrently, transfusion-associated CMV can be prevented. Several of the studies just cited show that CMV seronegativity can be established by performing a variety of assays. Freezing and deglycerolization of red cell components will prevent transmission. Leukocyte filtration although in the early stages is a method that will undoubtedly be shown to be efficacious. Lastly, selecting one method of prevention over another will have to do more with the impact on cost of those procedures and the supply. Not only will the CMV seroprevalence of the blood donor base affect supply, but increased patient transfusion requirements coming from groups other than neonates will increase demand. At the time the neonatal studies were performed and the transfusion standards established, bone marrow transplant pa-tients were not as numerous as they are today. From now on, issues of transfusion support for specific patients such as neonates will have to be considered as part of a shared supply of specialized CMV-seronegative or filtered blood components.

CMV Infection in the Donor

The next area to examine is the donor side of the transfusion-transmitted CMV issue. The basic question surrounding CMV negativity or positivity is whether or not the blood being transfused is infectious. Blood components have been labeled by serological assays that determine whether or not the donor has ever been infected with CMV. Like the other Herpes virus family members, CMV becomes latent following primary infection and later can reactivate; once the host is infected, he or she is always infected and antibody is detectable for life. Current serological assays cannot differentiate between those donors whose blood has antibody and no circulating virus and those whose blood has antibody and virus. Therefore, we must assume that all blood components from seropositive individuals are potentially infectious.

CMV transfusion studies indicate that only a subset of seropositive donors' blood components transmit CMV because only a small number of seronegative recipients of seropositive blood become infected with CMV. Additionally, not all transfusion recipients seem to be susceptible to CMV disease from TA-CMV infection. This outcome may be due to the nature of the blood component, to the immune response of the recipient or to a combination of both; the exact cause is not clearly understood.

Transmission Mechanisms

Two possible mechanisms for CMV transmission by blood transfusion have been proposed. The first is that infectious virus is transfused in a blood component collected from an actively infected but asymptomatic donor. The second is that the CMV genome in transfused cells from a latently infected asymptomatic donor becomes reactivated in the recipient. Depending on the stage of CMV infection in the donor, either mechanism could be operating. Additionally, the status of the host's immune response must be considered in evaluating which of these theoretical mechanisms is most likely. If infectious virus particles are present in the transfused blood, the effectiveness of the recipient's immune response will determine whether an infection becomes established. Alternatively, if only latent virus is present in the transfused blood, an additional trigger to reactivate the virus from donor cells may be necessary. The proposal has been made that leukocytes in the blood components provide allogeneic stimulation to the recipient's immune system, thus causing activation of the recipient's cells. Activation of the recipient's immune cells could lay the groundwork for the newly transmitted virus to become established. Whether viral pathogenicity plays a role in establishing this infection is unknown.

States of CMV Infection

To examine why all seropositive blood components do not transmit CMV, an understanding of the events following CMV infection of the donor is necessary; latency and reactivation are two characteristics of this virus that are critical. From general knowledge about latent viral infections in the human host, which mainly comes from studies of the other Herpes viruses, it is possible to hypothesize when antibody and virus occur during an infection. Unfortunately, there are little data to substantiate a model for CMV. However, using results from transfusion studies and from viral cultures of actively infected patients,[41] we can hypothesize that seropositive individuals do not stay in the same state of CMV infection over time. For example, some individuals may have been recently infected and have viremia, viruria and circulating IgM levels, indicating early stages of CMV infection. Other individuals may have antibody levels to certain viral antigens that are predominantly of the IgG class without detectable virus in either blood or urine, indicating a latent state of infection. Still another group may have circulating antibody to specific viral antigens and also have virus detectable by standard culture techniques. These three types of individuals could represent various stages of infection, including primary infection, latent infection and reactivated CMV infection, respectively, as illustrated in Fig 7-1.

The CMV antibody assays used clinically and in blood banks are produced using virus preparations consisting predominantly of late antigens (LA). IgG to LA develops soon after infection and persists indefinitely; thus, CMV seropositivity has been defined as the presence of IgG antibody to LA. However, antibodies can also be elicited against immediate early antigens (IE) and early antigens (EA), which are present in the nucleus, cytoplasm or membranes of CMV-infected cells. Pres-ence of IgG to CMV IE has been associated frequently, but not consistently, with primary or reactivated CMV infection and can last long after the cessation of viral shedding. The presence of antibody to EA has been reported to occur coincident with viral shedding in patients with primary CMV infec-

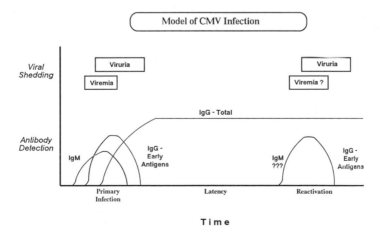

Figure 7-1. Model of CMV infection.

tions and had been associated with reactivated infection, with titers declining shortly after cessation of viral shedding. Since the presence of antibody to EA has been strongly associated both with the recent and ongoing viral replication in the host, its presence has been hypothesized to be a specific serological marker for actively infected, asymptomatic blood donors.

We evaluated 500 blood donors for presence of viruria, for presence of antibody to EA, and for seropositivity using ELISA and latex agglutination assays.[42] We concluded that while all serologic assays detected all viruric donors with 100% sensitivity, the assay for antibody to EA was more specific than ELISA or latex agglutination. The prevalence of viruria in our study of blood donors was low. Referring to Fig 7-1, if we hypothesize that these donors were experiencing reactivation and not having a primary CMV infection, then perhaps antibody to EA is a more valuable assay for selecting the asymptomatic individuals who are shedding virus. To determine if these donors are capable of transmitting CMV, these studies would need to be extended to evaluate the transfusion recipients.

Another question regarding use of serological testing to determine whether a blood donor is CMV-positive or -negative is whether transfusion of CMV antibody is passively protective for the recipient. Since use of hyperimmune globulin has been shown to diminish severity of disease in renal transplant recipients,[43] it seems reasonable to assume that antibody is somehow interfering with viral pathogenicity. This raises the question, "Is all CMV antibody the same?" Studies to evaluate whether antibodies to specific viral proteins are neutralizing and, therefore, potentially protective when passively transferred, would clarify the importance of these differences in antibody production. Although several neonatal transfusion study results have indicated the protective nature of antibody, further studies are needed to specifically define which CMV antibodies are protective. Additionally, while an asymptomatic, seropositive blood donor may transmit the virus at the same time antibody is being transfused, the use of red blood cell transfusion to provide passive immunization may not be the safest means.

Means for Prevention

Any significant increase in demand for CMV-negative blood components will be difficult to meet using current serologic procedures. Therefore, it is desirable to identify CMV-seropositive blood components that are not infectious. There is widespread agreement that not all CMV-seropositive blood components are capable of transmitting CMV, and that only a small subset of seropositive donors is infectious. Provision of CMV-negative blood components would be greatly facilitated by use of a rapid technique with the necessary sensitivity and specificity to identify infectious blood donors and distinguish those infectious from the many noninfectious seropositive do-nors.

Another technique that could be valuable for detecting the subset of infectious donors among the seropositives is the detection of CMV genome by amplification techniques such as polymerase chain reaction (PCR). The rationale supported by transfusion-associated CMV infections suggests that leukocytes circulating in the peripheral blood carry the genome of CMV. If this were true, then seropositive individuals should have levels of CMV genome detectable by PCR. Detection of CMV DNA in actively infected bone marrow transplant recipients, neonates and solid organ transplant recipients was easily demonstrable.[44-47] However, when peripheral blood samples from healthy seropositive individuals were assayed, no positive PCR results for CMV were found in one study[47] and two of three were positive in another.[46] At the Second International Cytomegalovirus Workshop held in San Diego, California in March of 1989, preliminary reports of PCR in asymptomatic CMV-seropositive individuals were presented. Among the groups reporting results of CMV PCR, no asymptomatic CMV-seropositive individuals had CMV genome detected by PCR and false-positive results in seronegative individuals were occasionally seen. Conclusions from this meeting have not been confirmed by publications to date. Although there is hope that some modification of gene amplification techniques will eventually become applicable for detection of CMV in seropositive individuals for identifying the subset of infectious seropositive donors, this is not at hand today.

An alternative approach to identifying CMV-infectious blood is to render blood noninfectious by leukocyte depletion or inactivation. Demonstration of the effectiveness of such approaches to reduction of CMV infectivity will not be possible by routine viral culture techniques, since with only one exception, multiple attempts to culture CMV from the blood of healthy blood donors have been unsuccessful.[17] Prospective clinical evaluations of the efficacy of measures to prevent transfusion-transmitted CMV require the detailed follow-up of large numbers of transfusion recipients because of the extremely low incidence of TA-CMV and the high prevalence of seropositivity in the recipient population. Furthermore, ethical considerations prevent the possibility of studying transmission in patient groups at risk for clinically significant CMV disease since transmission can be easily prevented by transfusing only CMV-seronegative blood. Therefore, a crystal ball and an evaluation of the current rapid pace of implementation of filtration methods prompt a prediction that molecular biological approaches for the detection of CMV nucleic acids may be employed in transfusion medicine as a means to detect effective depletion of the virus from cellular blood components after filtration rather than a rapid screening test for donor blood that would replace serology.

Blood Components and Treatments

The proven methods available for producing CMV-negative blood are serological screening and freezing/deglycerolization. For cost reasons, serological screening may have more advantages. Several studies comparing types of serological assays have been reported,[42,48-51] but of hemagglutination inhibition, complement fixation, ELISA, indirect immunofluorescence (IFA) and passive latex agglutination, only ELISA, IFA, and latex agglutination are readily available. Several investigators have compared assays and found latex agglutination assays to be the least expensive, most easily performed and most adaptable to the blood bank setting.[49-51] From a case report of two neonates with TA-CMV infections, the CMV latex agglutination assay was useful for retrospectively determining which of the donors' samples that had been mistakenly tested as negative were actually positive.[52] In addition to being a simple but accurate assay, the reagents are generally available at a price of just over one dollar. Although direct viral detection techniques are currently very useful in the clinical setting for detecting CMV in active disease, assays such as viral culture, viral antigen detection and viral nucleic acid detection by in situ hybridization or PCR are time-consuming, technically complex and expensive. Most importantly, these assays cannot dependably be used to detect CMV in latently infected asymptomatic individuals such as blood donors. Future development of any of these techniques into rapid diagnostic tools that could discriminate between active CMV shedding and latency in asymptomatic carriers would be very useful, but these assays are not presently developed to that point.

Red blood cells are the most frequently transfused component in hospitalized neonates. Often, these red cells are transfused in small aliquots provided in smaller than usual blood bags or from individual syringes. Many neonates may share a red cell component collected from one donor. The serological screening tests or leukocyte depletion methods referred to for neonatal transfusion are generally proposed to be used on packed red blood cells. Platelet transfusions are infrequently given to neonates. However, if CMV-seronegative packed red blood cells are given to a neonate to prevent CMV transmission, it would be prudent to also transfuse CMV-seronegative platelets. At this time, providing large volumes of CMV-seronegative platelets, as might be needed to support those neonatal intensive care units that employ a relatively new procedure (extracorporeal membrane oxygenation [ECMO]), could be difficult. Studies of CMV prevention using leukocyte depletion filters for platelet products are needed. Transfusion of fresh frozen plasma is a rare event in the neonatal intensive care unit; however, there should be no need to screen this component for CMV because there are no reports of CMV transmission by plasma. Transfusion of fresh red blood cells for neonates has been proposed as a reason for high transmission rates to neonates. The argument that fresher blood is more likely to transmit CMV than older blood is not an issue if red cell components are serologically screened or frozen. Transfusion studies have shown that deglycerolization prevents CMV transmission from red blood cells whether the original unit was CMV-seronegative or -seropositive. It seems wasteful to employ two prevention strategies for the same unit. However, it also seems prudent to use a combination of components that are least likely to transmit CMV infection once the need to prevent transmission has been assessed. As previously noted, CMV-seronegative red blood cells and CMV-seronegative platelets should be used together. One additional method that deserves comment is blood product irradiation. While the irradiation doses (1500 rad) are successfully em-ployed to prevent alloimmunization, this treatment does not affect infectivity of CMV.[53,54]

Rationale for CMV-Negative Blood Support

Applying what has been presented about CMV, its transmission by transfusion and the resulting disease in neonates raises several questions. What are the most reasonable, cost-effective, legal and ethical approaches for providing transfusion support for neonates? Which methodologies should be applied to which types of blood components? Which types of neonates should be transfused with which blood components at what cost? What follows is not an answer to these complicated questions, but rather a proposed rationale that supports use of CMV-negative blood components and prevents transmission of CMV to all low-birth-weight neonates.

Results of Clinical Studies

During the 1980's, many groups worldwide evaluated transfusion-transmitted CMV in hospitalized neonates by performing well-constructed, but difficult, lengthy and expensive clinical trials. Results from these studies have validated each other and should be the guide for decision-making. It is clear that the smaller, premature neonates have the highest morbidity and mortality. It is not clear whether the definition of "small" is <1200 g, <1250 g or <1500 g. Several avenues for prevention of CMV have been successfully implemented and there is agreement on how to prevent TA-CMV infection in seronegative neonates. Serological screening to exclude CMV-seropositive blood and freezing/deglycerolization of packed red blood cells are methods by which this can be accomplished. Results using filtration of red cells and platelets to prevent CMV transmission are extremely promising, but incomplete. There is no agreement about what degree of severity of disease is sufficient to justify what cost for prevention. In part, this stems from unchangeable circumstances that dictate how health-care costs are divided and funding appropriated. There also is no general agreement on which prevention procedures are the most cost-effective for each blood supplier and patient population. This should not be a problem if transfusion standards can remain flexible. Obviously, blood centers have different constraints and those supporting bone marrow transplant units or neonatal intensive care units that provide ECMO have different blood supply management problems than those that do not.

Policy Dilemmas

What all of these studies cannot answer clearly is the nagging question of blood support for seropositive neonates. Several points form the rationale for justifying provision of CMV negative blood components to these neonates as well as the sero-negative neonates. The first is that reinfection with a new strain of CMV is possible when seropositive units of blood are transfused. Presence of circulating antibody does not prevent infection with a new strain of CMV.[55] Second, serologic testing of the mother or infant may inadvertently identify a seronegative baby as falsely seropositive. Two such cases have been described by Logan.[52] In these cases, inadequacy of serologic testing and the time of performance of the study can be cited as the causes of this problem. However, there are many laboratories throughout the world performing relatively unstandardized tests, and it is conceivable that this kind of situation could be repeated. The third point is actually the first one historically. Adler has stated that as seropositive neonates become seronegative through depletion of their passive maternal antibody by frequent blood collection during hospitalization, they may become more susceptible to infection and disease the same way that seronegative neonates do. Tegtmeier has argued that seropositive infants become seronegative even faster when only seronegative blood components are transfused. Although there is clear documentation that seropositive neonates do become seronegative over extended periods of hospitalization, both sides of this issue remain controversial. However, the first two points, reinfection and possible inadequacy of serological testing, can be used as support for providing seronegative blood to these neonates. Lastly, a case can be made that a single supply of blood for a neonatal intensive care unit simplifies transfusion logistics in this setting. Potential for mixing blood supplies would be eliminated, as well as most efficiently using a limited supply of blood by sharing one unit for several infants.

Blood providers currently go through extraordinary efforts to provide blood for neonatal transfusions. We specially recruit repeat donors who are group O, sickle-cell negative and then select those who have taken no medications, particularly aspirin. We collect these donors' blood in anticoagulant solutions without additives such as mannitol or adenine, which could be injurious to an immature neonatal liver. In addition, the blood we collect for neonates is placed in special collection containers such as quad/quint packs to provide convenient small volumes for the nursery. Alternatively, blood is sometimes collected in larger containers, then connected by sterile connecting devices to transfer blood to specialized packs or syringe arrangements. We then rapidly transport these units so that the nursery receives fresh blood that can be transfused within 10 days of collection.

There is a proven ability to continually supply this specialized red cell component for neonates. Adding CMV serological screening to the front end of this procedure is workable unless the seroprevalence of the donor population is very high. For geographic areas where CMV seroprevalence is high, the issue of sufficient supply is a problem. Although cost issues surrounding filtration techniques still need to be resolved, the rapid development of efficient leukocyte filtration techniques, therefore, may be the technology of the future that allows provision of CMV-negative blood components in high sero-prevalence areas.

Establishment of any single policy regarding neonatal transfusion and CMV transmission could cause potential problems for either the seronegative neonate or the seropositive neonate. If passively transferred antibody is indeed a protective measure that decreases severity of CMV disease in seropositive neonates as first proposed by Yeager's studies,[56] then a policy providing only CMV-seronegative blood to all neonates could place seropositive infants at some disadvantage. Noninfectious sources of this same antibody are available by use of fresh frozen plasma or intravenous gamma globulin preparations. Therefore, as with seronegative neonates, some effort and increased cost to the blood providers and to the health-care delivery systems seem warranted to prevent transmission of new CMV infection to individuals who already may be infected, even though this phenomenon is not yet completely understood.

Summary

In summary, provision of CMV-negative blood for neonates requiring transfusion is a responsibility of the blood bank community today. By doing this, transfusion-associated CMV infections can be prevented in seronegative neonates and untested neonates. In addition, other CMV strains and unknown related infection in seropositive neonates can be prevented. Although this represents small numbers of infections and perhaps eliminates only a very small amount of disease, there is sufficient documentation of transfusion transmission to require such action. Moreover, there are insufficient data on the sequelae of CMV infection that sometimes manifest later in childhood. It appears that infection with CMV is better handled later in life in a host with a more mature immune system than during the perinatal period. Studies of the natural transmission of CMV clearly report that young children, in particular those in day-care settings, readily become infected with CMV. However, studies suggest that these children remain asymptomatic. Clearly, we are not preventing CMV transmission forever, but simply moving it from an iatrogenic source into the realm of natural transmission.

References

1. Rook AH. Interactions of cytomegalovirus with the human immune system. J Infect Dis 1988;10:S460.
2. Apperley JF, Goldman JM. Cytomegalovirus: Biology, clinical features and methods for diagnosis. Bone Marrow Transplant 1988;3:253-64.
3. Schrier RD, Nelson JA, Oldstone MBA. Detection of human cytomegalovirus in peripheral blood lymphocytes in a natural infection. Science 1985;230:1048-51.
4. Kaariainen L, Klemola E, Paloheimo J. Rise of cytomegalovirus antibodies in an infectious-mononucleosis-like syndrome after transfusion. Br Med J 1966;1:1270-2.
5. Foster KM, Jack I. A prospective study of the role of cytomegalovirus in post-transfusion mononucleosis. N Engl J Med 1969;280:1311-16.
6. Hanshaw JB. A new cytomegalovirus syndrome. Am J Dis Child 1979;133:475-6.
7. Kumar A, Nankervis GA, Cooper AR, et al. Acquisition of cytomegalovirus infection in infants following exchange transfusion: A prospective study. Transfusion 1980;20:327-31.
8. Benson JWT, Bodden SJ, Tobin J. Cytomegalovirus and blood transfusion in neonates. Arch Dis Child 1979;54:538-41.
9. Ballard RA, Drew WL, Hufnagle KG, Riedel PA. Acquired cytomegalovirus infections in preterm infants. Am J Dis Child 1979;133:482-5.
10. Yeager AS. Transfusion-acquired cytomegalovirus infection in newborn infants. Am J Dis Child 1974;128:478-83.
11. Yeager AS, Grumet FC, Hafleigh EB, et al. Prevention of transfusion-acquired cytomegalovirus infections in newborn infants. J Pediatr 1981;98:281-87.
12. Adler SP, Chandrika T, Lawrence L, Baggett J. Cytomegalovirus infections in neonates acquired by blood transfusions. Pediatr Infect Dis 1983;2:114-18.
13. Schmidt P, ed. Standards for blood banks and transfusion services. 11th ed. Arlington, VA: American Association of Blood Banks, 1984:27-8.
14. Adler SP. Transfusion-associated cytomegalovirus infections. Rev Infect Dis 1983;5:977-93.
15. Adler SP. Neonatal cytomegalovirus infections due to blood. CRC Crit Rev Clin Lab Sci 1986;23:1-14.
16. Tegtmeier GE. Cytomegalovirus infection as a complication of blood transfusion. Semin Liver Dis 1986;6:82-95.

17. Tegtmeier GE. Posttransfusion cytomegalovirus infections. Arch Pathol Lab Med 1989;113:236-45.
18. Ho M. Cytomegalovirus biology and infection. New York: Plenum Medical Book Company, 1982.
19. Rawls WE, Wong CL, Blajchman M, et al. Neonatal cytomegalovirus infections: The relative role of neonatal blood transfusion and maternal exposure. Clin Invest Med 1984; 7:13-19.
20. Griffin MP, O'Shea M, Brazy JE, et al. Cytomegalovirus infection in a neonatal intensive care unit blood transfusion practices and incidence of infection. Am J Dis Child 1988;142:1188.
21. Lamberson HV, McMillan JA, Weiner LB, et al. Prevention of transfusion-associated cytomegalovirus (CMV) infection in neonates by screening blood donors for IgM to CMV. J Infect Dis 1988;157:820-3.
22. Preiksaitis JK, Brown L, McKenzie M. Transfusion-acquired cytomegalovirus infection in neonates. Transfusion 1988;28:205-9.
23. Tegtmeier GE. The use of cytomegalovirus-screened blood in neonates. Transfusion 1988; 28:201-03.
24. Gilbert GL, Hayes K, Hudson IL, James J. Prevention of transfusion-acquired cytomegalovirus infection in infants by blood filtration to remove leucocytes. Lancet 1989;1: 1228-31.
25. Bhumbra NA, Lewandowski P, Lau P, et al. Evaluation of a prescreening blood donor program for prevention of perinatal transfusion-acquired cytomegalovirus (CMV) infection. J Perinat Med 1988;16:127.
26. Weston PJ, Farmer K, Croxson MC, Ramirez AM. Morbidity from acquired cytomegalovirus infection in a neonatal intensive care unit. Aust Paediatr J 1989;25:138-42.
27. Adler SP, Lawrence LT, Baggett J, et al. Prevention of transfusion-associated cytomegalovirus infection in very low-birth-weight infants using frozen blood and donors seronegative for cytomegalovirus. Transfusion 1984;24: 333-5.
28. Brady MT, Milam JD, Anderson DC, et al. Use of deglycerolized red blood cells to prevent posttransfusion infection with cytomegalovirus in neonates. J Infect Dis 1984; 150:334-9.
29. Taylor BJ, Jacobs RF, Baker RL, et al. Frozen deglycerolyzed blood prevents transfusion-acquired cytomegalovirus infections in neonates. Pediatr Infect Dis 1986;5: 188-91.

30. Simon T, Johnson J, Koffler H, et al. Impact of previously frozen deglycerolized red blood cells on cytomegalovirus transmission to newborn infants. Plasma Ther Transfus Technol 1987;8:51-6.
31. Demmler GJ, Brady MT, Bijou H, et al. Posttransfusion cytomegalovirus infection in neonates: Role of saline-washed red blood cells. J Pediatr 1986;108:762-5.
32. Luban NLC, Williams AE, MacDonald MG, et al. Low incidence of acquired cytomegalovirus infection in neonates transfused with washed red blood cells. Am J Dis Child 1987;141:416-19.
33. Beneke JS, Tegtmeier GE, Alter HJ, et al. Relation of titers of antibodies to CMV in blood donors to the transmission of cytomegalovirus infection. J Infect Dis 1984;150:883-8.
34. Bowden RA, Sayers MH, Cays M, Slicher SJ. The role of blood product filtration in the prevention of transfusion associated cytomegalovirus (CMV) infection after marrow transplant. (abstract) Transfusion 1989;29S:57S.
35. Wilhelm JA, Matter L, Schopfer K. The risk of transmitting cytomegalovirus to patients receiving blood transfusions. J Infect Dis 1986;154:169-71.
36. Preiksaitis JK, Brown L, McKenzie M. The risk of cytomegalovirus infection in seronegative transfusion recipients not receiving exogenous immunosuppression. J Infect Dis 1988;157:523-9.
37. Gjesdal K, Orstavik I, Fagerhol M, et al. Blood donor selection can prevent cytomegalovirus infection after open heart surgery. Eur Heart J 1987;8:378-83.
38. Mackinnon S, Burnett AK, Crawford RI, et al. Seronegative blood products prevent primary cytomegalovirus infection after bone marrow transplantation. J Clin Pathol 1988;41:948-50.
39. Bowden RA, Sayers M, Gleaves CA, et al. Cytomegalovirus-seronegative blood components for the prevention of primary cytomegalovirus infection after marrow transplantation. Transfusion 1987;27:478-81.
40. Verdonck LF, de Graan-Hentzen YCE, Dekker AW, et al. Cytomegalovirus seronegative platelets and leukocyte-poor red blood cells from random donors can prevent primary cytomegalovirus infection after bone marrow transplantation. Bone Marrow Transplant 1987;2:7-78.
41. Feletti C, Musiani M, Bonomini V. Early diagnosis of cytomegalovirus infection in renal transplantation. Proc Eur Dial Transplant Assoc 1980;17:473-7.
42. Lentz EB, Dock NL, McMahon CA, et al. Detection of antibody to cytomegalovirus-induced early antigens and

comparison with four serologic assays and presence of viruria in blood donors. J Clin Microbiol 1988;26:133-5.

43. Snydman DR, Werner BG, Heinze-Lacey B, et al. Use of cytomegalovirus immune globulin to prevent cytomegalovirus disease in renal-transplant recipients. N Engl J Med 1987;317:1049-54.

44. Demmler GJ, Buffone GJ, Schimbor CM, May RA. Detection of cytomegalovirus in urine from newborns by using polymerase chain reaction DNA amplification. J Infect Dis 1988;158:1177-84.

45. Olive DM, Simsek M, Al-Mufti S. Polymerase chain reaction assay for detection of human cytomegalovirus. J Clin Microbiol 1989;27:1238-42.

46. Cassol SA, Poon M, Pal R, et al. Primer-mediated enzymatic amplification of cytomegalovirus (CMV) DNA: Application to the early diagnosis of CMV infection in marrow transplant recipients. J Clin Invest 1989;83:1109-15.

47. Shibata D, Martin WJ, Appleman MD, et al. Detection of cytomegalovirus DNA in peripheral blood of patients infected with human immunodeficiency virus. J Infect Dis 1988;158:1185-92.

48. Beckwith DG, Halstead DC, Alpaugh K, et al. Comparison of a latex agglutination test with five other methods for determining the presence of antibody against cytomegalovirus. J Clin Microbiol 1985;21:328-31.

49. Taswell HF, Reisner RK, Rabe DE, et al. Comparison of three methods for detecting antibody to cytomegalovirus. Transfusion 1986;26:285-9.

50. Feng CS, Williams IB, Gohd RS, Causey AP. A comparison of four commercial test kits for detection of cytomegalovirus antibodies in blood donors. Transfusion 1986;26:203-4.

51. Klinedinst AF, Baldwin ML, Ness PM. Detection of cytomegalovirus antibody in stored blood products using latex agglutination. Transfusion 1988;28:563-5.

52. Logan S, Barbara J, Kovar I. Cytomegalovirus screened blood for neonatal intensive care units. Arch Dis Child 1989; 63:753-7.

53. Chou S, Kim DY, Norman DI. Transmission of cytomegalovirus by pretransplant leukocyte transfusions in renal transplant candidates. J Infect Dis 1987;155:565-7.

54. Winston DJ, Ho WG, Howell CL, et al. Cytomegalovirus infections associated with leukocyte transfusions. Ann Intern Med 1980;93:671-4.

55. Chandler SH, Handsfield HH, McDougall JK. Isolation of multiple strains of cytomegalovirus from women attending

a clinic for sexually transmitted diseases. J Infect Dis 1987;155:655-60.

56. Yeager AS, Palumbo PE, Malachowski N, et al. Sequelae of maternally derived cytomegalovirus infections in premature infants. J Pediatr 1983;102:918-22.

Index

(Italicized page numbers indicate tables or figures.)

A

AIDS. *See* Immunodeficiency syndrome, acquired

Alloimmunization
Class I, 16-17, 18, 37
Class II, 17, 37, 48
incidence, 36
mechanisms, 17-*19*-20
prevention, 14, 22-24, 35-*39*-40
UV irradiation, 47-49

Anamnestic response, leukocyte depleted blood components, 23

Anemia, aplastic
GVHD, 43, 61, *64*
leukocyte-depleted blood components — CON, 13-32
leukocyte-depleted blood components — PRO, 33-55

B

B lymphocytes, responses, 18

Birth weight, low
CMV infection, 116-117, 118-119
CMV-negative transfusions, 146

Blood components, CMV-"safe," 144-145
methods, 122
neonatal recipients, 117, 120

Blood components, leukocyte-depleted, 13-22
leukocyte-poor, vs, 14-15
quality control, 21-22
recommendations, 26
routine use, 22-25, 26

Blood components, leukocyte-poor
benefits, 35-43
leukocyte-depleted, vs, 14-15

Buffy coat, purified platelets, 38

C

Cardiac surgery
GVHD, 60, *65*
See also Transplantation

Cellselect, 46

Chemotherapy, leukemia, 35

Cytomegalic inclusion disease (CID), 84-*85*

Cytomegalovirus, 81
activation, 83-84
antibody prevalence, 103
characteristics, 131-133
molecular biology, 82-84
prevalence, 132
screening, 120, 143
transfusion issues, 133
transmission mechanisms, 109, 140
virus-cell association, 132-133

Cytomegalovirus infection, 2-3, 49, 103-104
allograft recipient, 114
BMT, allogeneic, 87-89
BMT, autologous, 89-*90*-93
congenital, 84-*85*
future, 97-98
GVHD, 88
immunocompetence, 114
manifestations, 84-*85*
non-transfusion-acquired, 113-114
pneumonia, interstitial, 87-89
policy dilemmas, 146-148
posttransplantation, organ, 87-95
prevention, 7, 13, 24-25, 26, 95-98
primary, 84
secondary, 84
seronegative donors, use of 81-102
feasibility, 96-97
necessity, 95-96
perinatal patient, 103-130, 131-153

Cytomegalovirus infection, neonatal, 104
donor, 139-140
donor factors, geographic, 115-116
donor factors that influence risk, 110-111
geographic variability, 115-117
historical perspective, 104-*106*-107, 133-140
incidence, 105-*106*, *135*
leukocytes, 107, 109
morbidity and mortality, 107, *108*

155

pathogenesis model, 112-113
prevention, 136-*137*-139, 142-
144
recipient factors, geographic,
116-117
recipient factors that influence
risk, 111-112
seronegative components,
alternatives to, 120-123
indications for, 120, *121*,
145-148
seronegative donors — CON,
103-130
seronegative donors — PRO,
131-153

D
Dendritic cells, 19, 20-21
DR antigen, 20, 26

E
ECMO. *See* Membrane oxygena-
tion, extracorporeal
Erypur, 4, 45-46
Febrile reactions. *See* Transfusion
reactions, nonhemolytic febrile
Filters, third-generation, 14
Filters, fourth-generation, 98

G
Glomerulonephropathy, CMV infection, 92
Graft-vs-host disease, posttransfusion (GVHD-PT), 1-2
anemia, aplastic, 61, *64*
BMT, 42-43
cardiac surgery, 60, *65*, 70-71
CMV infection, 88
historical perspective, 58-61
haplotype commonality, 66-67,
71
immunodeficiency syndrome,
61, *64*
irradiation of blood components, 57-80
leukemia, 61, *64*
lymphoma, 61, *63*
malignancies, 60, *65*, 66, 70
manifestations, 57-58, 61
mortality, 61
newborns, 60, *62*, 66
predisposing factors, 66-67
prevention, 13, 58, 67-70
risk, 61-*62-63-64-65*
Granulocytes, HLA distribution, 16
Granulocytes, polymorphonuclear,
function after collection, 15-16

Granulocyte transfusions, 88
neonates, 119

H
Herpes viruses, 82-83
Histocompatibility complex, major
Class I, 16-18, 37
Class II, 17, 37, 48
HLA antigen, 37
Class I, 16-17, 18, 37
Class II, 17, 37, 48
distribution in blood, 16-17

I
IgM
CMV-negative, 137-138
CMV-specific, 110
Immunocompetence, CMV infec-
tion, 114
Immunodeficiency syndrome, ac-
quired, GVHD-PT, 66
Immunosuppression, transfusion-
induced, *2*-5, 83
Imugard IG500, 4, 14, 45
Interleukin-1 (IL-1), 18-*19*, 48
Irradiation, gamma
adverse effects, 68-69
blood component function, 67-
68
GVHD prevention, 67-69, 71
Irradiation, UV, 47-49, 69-70

L
Leukemia
BMT, 42
chemotherapy, 35
GVHD, 42, 61, *64*
leukocyte-depleted blood components, 13-32, 33-55
Leukocyte depletion, 3-5, 69
centrifugation, 44
CMV infection, 143
filtration, 4-*5*, 44, 45-47
methods, 44-47
timing, 47
Leukocytes, 1-2
content in blood components,
22, 34-35
function after collection, 16
HLA distribution, 16
number transfused, 23-24
Leukocytes, donor
blood components, 15-16
HLA alloimmunization, 17-*19*-
20
HLA antigen distribution, 16-17
importance, quantitative, 20-21

Lymphocytotoxic antibody, 36, 37

M

Membrane oxygenation, extracorporeal, 120
8-Methoxypsoralen (8-MOP), 18, *19*
Miropoor L, 45
Monocytes, 19, 20-21
    CMV, 109
Mononucleosis, heterophile negative, 84-*85*

N

Neoplasms, transfusion, 2-3
Newborns
    GVHD, 60, *62*
    See also Cytomegalovirus infection
NHFTR. *See* Transfusion reactions, nonhemolytic febrile

P

Pall PL100, 45, 98
Pall RC100, 4, *5*, 98
Plasma, HLA distribution, 16
Platelet concentrates
    HLA-matched, 26
    leukocyte contamination, 15
    UV-irradiated, 47-48
Platelets
    CMV infection, 90
    CMV negative, 145
    filters, 45-46
    hemostatic effectiveness, 46-47
    HLA distribution, 16
    purified, 37-38
Platelet transfusion, 37-38
    alloimmunization, 35
    prevention of refractoriness to, 24
Pneumonia, interstitial
    CMV-induced, 87-89
    risk factors, 87-88
Polymerase chain reaction
    CMV detection, 109, 121, 143
Polymorphonuclear cells, CMV, 109
Post-pump syndrome, 81-82

R

Red blood cells
    CMV-negative, 145
    filters, 46-47
    HLA distribution, 16
Red blood cells, deglycerolized, 136

Red blood cells, leukocyte-depleted, 1-11
    benefits, 7
    cost, 7
    thalassemia patients, 5, *6*
Red blood cells, saline-washed,
    CMV infection, 122
Refractoriness to platelets
    leukocyte-depleted, 24
    leukocyte-poor, 38-*39*-40
    UV irradiation, 49

S

Sepacell PL, 45
Sepacell R500, 4, *5*, 14

T

T lymphocytes, 37
    depletion pretransfusion, 69-70
    response, 19-20
Thalassemia, leukocyte-depleted
    red cell transfusion, 5, *6*
Transplantation, bone marrow
    allogeneic, and CMV infection, 87-89
    autologous, and CMV infection, 89-*90*-93
    CMV infection, 138
    leukocyte-poor blood components, 42-44
Transplantation, cardiac, CMV infection, *94*-95, 138
Transplantation, kidney
    CMV infection, 92
    seroconversion, 92-*93*
Transplantation, liver, CMV infection, *94*-95
Transplantation, solid organ, *94*
    CMV infection, 114
Tumors, solid, GVHD, 60, *65*
Transfusion effect, 2
Transfusion reactions, nonhemolytic febrile, 1, 3
    leukocyte-depleted blood component, 13-14, 25, 44
    leukocyte-poor blood components, 40-42
    prevention, 7, 13-14, 25, 40-42
    techniques, 14, 26

U-V

Ultipor SQ40S, 4, *5*, 14
UV-A irradiation, 18, *19*
Viruses. *See* Cytomegalovirus